George Winston Smith

Medicines for the Union Army
The United States Army Laboratories During the Civil War

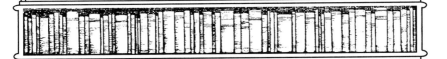

More pre-publication
REVIEWS, COMMENTARIES, EVALUATIONS . . .

"Smith has presented a detailed history of the U.S. Army's development of two pharmaceutical manufacturing and testing laboratories during the Civil War and of the men involved. The need for such facilities was in response to problems with foreign supplies, domestic drug companies, brokers, high prices, and limited supplies of medications. In addition to excellent notes and references, the methods and systems required to overcome a number of difficulties in manufacturing, packaging, and politics are presented in a clear, sequential fashion."

Jack D. Welsh, MD
David Ross Boyd Professor Emeritus,
University of Oklahoma

"The two million men in the Union army suffered six million reported episodes of illness, generating an enormous demand for medicines. Speculators and profiteers drove up the prices of raw and finished pharmaceuticals, even as the federal government teetered on the edge of bankruptcy.

In an almost-forgotten success story, the U.S. Army created two pharmaceutical manufacturing laboratories; their dedication and innovative technical brilliance saved thousands of lives and (in today's money) 40 million dollars. This never-before-told story is a significant addition to our understanding of America's great conflict."

Thomas P. Lowry, MD
Author of five books on the Civil War

"Professor Smith has done more than a credible job by providing a rare insight into the medicines used during the Civil War and how they were obtained. His detailed accounts of the development of the little-known Army laboratories and the efforts of the surgeon general's office to curb the high cost of medicines during that war are a major contribution to the overall knowledge of that era. The book provides a treasure trove of data for the serious researcher and Civil War writer. A very major effort showing a fine eye for detail and a clear presentation of the information. Well done!"

Robert E. Denney, BS, MS
Author,
Past President,
Civil War Round Table,
Washington, D.C.

Medicines
for the Union Army
The United States
Army Laboratories
During the Civil War

PHARMACEUTICAL PRODUCTS PRESS
Pharmaceutical Heritage:
Pharmaceutical Care Through History

Mickey C. Smith, PhD
Dennis B. Worthen, PhD
Senior Editors

Laboratory on the Nile: A History of the Wellcome Tropical Research Laboratories by Patrick F. D'Arcy

America's Botanico-Medical Movements: Vox Populi by Alex Berman and Michael A. Flannery

Medicines for the Union Army: The United States Army Laboratories During the Civil War by George Winston Smith

Pharmaceutical Education in the Queen City: 150 Years of Service, 1850-2000 by Michael A. Flannery and Dennis B. Worthen

Medicines
for the Union Army
The United States Army Laboratories During the Civil War

George Winston Smith

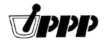

Pharmaceutical Products Press®
An Imprint of The Haworth Press, Inc.
New York • London • Oxford

Published by

Pharmaceutical Heritage Editions, a series from Pharmaceutical Products Press®, an imprint of The Haworth Press, Inc., 10 Alice Street, Binghamton, NY 13904-1580

Cover design by Monica L. Seifert.

Library of Congress Cataloging-in-Publication Data

Smith, George Winston.
    Medicines for the Union Army : the United States Army laboratories during the Civil War / George Winston Smith.
        p.   cm.
    Originally published: Madison, Wsc. : American Institute of the History of Pharmacy, 1962.
    Includes bibliographical references and index.
    ISBN 0-7890-0946-3 (hard : alk. paper) — ISBN 0-7890-0947-1 (soft : alk. paper)
    1. United States—History—Civil War, 1861-1865—Medical care. 2. Medicine, Military—Research—United States—History—19th century. 3. Laboratories—United States—History—19th century. 4. United States. Army—History—Civil War, 1861-1865. I. Title.

E621 .S66 2000
973.7'75—dc21

00-031924

CONTENTS

ABOUT THE AUTHOR

George Winston Smith served as Professor of History at the University of New Mexico. His other books include *Henry C. Carey and American Sectional Conflict,* and with co-author Charles Judah, *Life in the North During the Civil War* and *Unchosen.* Smith and Judah also co-edited *Chronicles of the Gringos: The U.S. Army in the Mexican War—Accounts of Eyewitnesses and Combatants.*

Foreword

Nearly forty years have passed since the American Institute of the History of Pharmacy first published George Winston Smith's classic *Medicines for the Union Army*. It remains the authority on the subject. When The Haworth Press approached us concerning a reprint, we were thrilled at the prospect. *Medicines* has been out of print for many years and we are tired of telling prospective readers that fact. Moreover, the editors at The Haworth Press have done an excellent job bringing the language into a more contemporary style with small stylistic changes that make the book more accessible for today's readers.

In 1962, Glenn Sonnedecker, then director of the American Institute of the History of Pharmacy, said this about Smith's work:

> A century ago many pharmacists were carrying musket or saber or pestle onto the battlefield; drug supplies were becoming uncertain; prices were beginning to rise. The American Civil War affected pharmacy also by spurring the development of pharmaceutical manufacturing, as wars have done before and since. Less well known is that the bloody vastness of the pharmaceutical demand was not met by private enterprise alone. The war's end would close a venture into government drug manufacturing just as firmly as it would close a period of American history. An anachronism of their time, the Union Laboratories gained a place . . . largely because of undisciplined (sometimes chaotic) conditions in the pharmaceutical market, profession and industry, coupled with sudden wartime exigencies.

William Procter, Jr., later affectionately termed a "father of American pharmacy," said of the events that swirled about him (1863): "The actual history of the medical supplies of the U.S. Army during the present rebellion, will furnish an interesting chapter in the history of the war would it ever be faithfully written."

According to Sonnedecker, Smith succeeded in writing that "interesting chapter" with *Medicines for the Union Army.** The book's attention to scholarship will no doubt keep readers informed about this subject for decades to come.

Gregory J. Higby, Director
American Institute of the History of Pharmacy
Madison, Wisconsin

---

*Glenn Sonnedecker, "Foreword," in George Winston Smith, *Medicines for the Union Army* (Madison, WI: American Institute of the History of Pharmacy, 1962), p. v.

Acknowledgments

It is impossible to list all of the librarians whose helpfulness and efficiency made the research easier. Among them, however, I should like to mention Miss Winifred Sewell, then Librarian at The Squibb Institute for Medical Research Library, New Brunswick, New Jersey; Mrs. Elizabeth W. Johnson, Librarian, Philadelphia College of Pharmacy and Science Library; Miss Mildred E. Blake, Librarian, Lovelace Foundation for Medical Education and Research, Albuquerque; Mr. Charles Roos, Documents Librarian, National Library of Medicine; Miss Ruth H. Davis, Library of the Wisconsin State Historical Society; Miss Genevieve Porterfield, Mr. Charles W. Warren, and Mr. Robert B. Harness, all of the University of New Mexico library. In addition, I wish to thank my friend, Mr. Buford Rowland, of the National Archives, Washington, D.C., for the encouragement and cooperation he gave to me. Dean Roy Bowers, when he was Dean of the College of Pharmacy, University of New Mexico, had much to do with establishing in that university's library a collection of source materials (some of the volumes coming from his personal library) that made this study possible. Mr. William H. Owings was both skillful and resourceful in preparing most of the prints for illustrations.

The research was partially financed by two grants from the Social Science Research Council, these grants being made for a wider study of the North during the Civil War of which this is a part. This book, however, neither could have been carried beyond its initial stages nor completed without the kind help, inspiration, and support given to me in many ways by Dr. Glenn Sonnedecker, Director of the American Institute of the History of

Pharmacy. My debt to him is immeasurable. I also wish to express my appreciation to Dr. Ernst W. Stieb, Secretary of the Institute, for his courteous and friendly aid. My wife, Helen M. Smith, was my constant co-worker at every stage.

George Winston Smith, 1962

Chapter 1

The Medical Purveying System and Its Problems

In the final months of the Civil War, as the Army of the Potomac besieged Petersburg and Sherman made ready at Savannah for his devastating sweep northward through the Carolinas, William Procter Jr., the "father of American pharmacy," reflected upon the quantities of medicines that had been supplied to the Union army. He concluded that never before, not even in the wars of Europe, had military pharmaceutical operations reached such tremendous proportions.[1] Procter could have elaborated by noting that the number of casualties might have been as large or even larger in previous European wars, but that the degree of neglect had always exceeded the amount of attention given to the sick and wounded.

Even in France, where military medicine had developed to a high degree of perfection during the reign of Louis XIV, the military hospitals that "le roi soleil" ordered to be erected were chiefly used for the enrichment of the civilian entrepreneurs who administered them.[2] Frederick the Great permitted Prussian executioners to treat the ulcers, fractures, and wounds of his men, and waged his Silesian campaign with his army sadly deficient in surgeons.[3] In spite of the brilliant services of Dominique-Jean Larrey, the greatest military surgeon and administrator of his time, the sick and wounded of Napoleon's army often were left to die without medical care on the field or were carried into barns or other nearby structures, then abandoned.[4] Compared to the 218,952

1

British soldiers who were hospitalized during the Crimean War,[5] far more than a million cases were treated in the 192 general hospitals of the United States Army during the Civil War.[6]

Concern for the sick and wounded of the federal armies was self-evident in the medical statistics. There were more than 6,000,000 reported cases of disease, and another 500,000 men who suffered battle wounds, accidents, and other injuries.[7] Among the white troops alone (statistics for Negro* troops covered only the period from July 1, 1863 to June 30, 1866), there were 1,213,685 cases of malaria; 139,638 cases of typhoid fever; 67,763 cases of measles; 61,202 cases of pneumonia; 73,382 cases of syphilis; and 109,397 cases of gonorrhea between May 1, 1861 and June 30, 1866.[8] Any discussion of these figures in terms of modern achievements would immediately disclose the limitations of medical science in the Civil War era; preventive medicine was limited to the prophylactic use of quinine and the empirical application of a few disinfectants, without any real understanding of the germ theory of disease. Despite the advances that came out of the experiences of the war, especially in surgery and neurology, as Reasoner has said, by modern standards "much of the theory and practice was still wrong."[9] But in the evolution of the army's Medical Department from incompetence to general efficiency, in the vastly improved organization and supply system fashioned by William A. Hammond, Jonathan Letterman, the medical purveyors, and others who worked under the surgeon general, and in the general environment, which was created for healing and recuperation, there was evidence of a great achievement. Not only was the mortality rate less than in any previous war, but the ratio of deaths from disease compared to battle deaths was lower among the northern troops than in any war before then.[10]

---

*The term "Negro" was common usage at the time this book was written and is not in any way intended as derogatory.—Ed.

The Civil War was a war of superlatives, one that involved millions of combatants, mountainous quantities of material, and an unprecedented power in its weapons to maim and kill. It also was fought during the "heroic age" of medicine by a generation of believers in the healing power of a complex array of drugs, administered in massive dosage.[11] When the standard supply table of the United States Army was fully revised in 1862 to meet the needs of the sick and wounded, it embraced "a more liberal supply of articles and drugs than [was] furnished to any army in the world."[12] No less than 131 distinct varieties of materia medica and pharmaceutical preparations from the supply table went through the Medical Department's major purveying depots to the armies.[13]

In quantity, these drugs varied from 1,232 ounces of strychnine to 539,712 pounds of magnesium sulfate.[14] The total issue of opium preparations (including powdered opium, powdered opium and ipecac, tincture of opium, and Camphorated Tincture of Opium) was 2,841,596 ounces, and, in addition, 442,926 dozen opium pills. The medical purveyors sent forward 987,687 ounces of ether (Aether Fortior); 1,588,066 ounces of chloroform; 1,688,943 ounces of sweet spirit of nitre (Spiritus Aetheris Nitrici); and of the various cinchona products, 2,072,040 ounces.[15] As an emetic and diaphoretic, ipecac had been superseded to a degree by calomel earlier in the nineteenth century, but it was once again in demand during the war,[16] especially for dysentery,[17] in three forms. As a fluid extract, as a powder, and in combination with opium, 1,005,779 ounces of it went to the troops.[18] A number of fluid extracts, first introduced in the fourth revision of the United States Pharmacopoeia (1863), were issued: ipecac, 268,936 ounces; cinchona, 544,110 ounces; and ginger, 607,940 ounces.[19] Among the other preparations supplied in large quantities were copaiba (1,292,129 ounces), powdered acacia (1,050,580 ounces), extract of licorice (818,485 ounces), tincture of ferric chloride (690,692 ounces), Hoffmann's anodyne (367,807 ounces), and camphor

(569,485 ounces). The armies also received 2,430,785 quart bottles of medical whiskey.[20]

The great variety and enormous volume of medical supplies reached the Union armies only through a difficult trial and error process that brought significant changes in the Medical Department of the United States Army. From almost every standpoint the army medical system was inadequate to meet the unprecedented situation created by the outbreak of hostilities at Fort Sumter. The backlog of supplies at the New York City purveying depot was small, the War Department lacked adequate funds to buy more of them in the market,[21] the manufacturers of pharmaceutical preparations (with the exception of Edward R. Squibb and a few others) were unprepared to meet the government's requisitions without delays,[22] and the administration of the Medical Bureau by Surgeon General Clement A. Finley and other conservative old-school officers—who still thought essentially in terms of a regular army of 13,000 men—revealed little imagination in dealing with the new medical problems.[23]

Nevertheless, in the summer of 1861, a revised edition of the *Regulations of the United States Army* contained a medical supply table that changed the quantities of medicines recommended for the army.[24] After Brigadier General William Alexander Hammond became surgeon general in 1862, a thorough revision of the supply table accompanied other innovations in the purveying system. At his direction, a board composed of surgeon Richard S. Satterlee, United States Army medical purveyor in New York City; surgeon R. O. Abbott, United States Army; and Edward R. Squibb, convened to discuss and recommend alterations in the supply table.[25] Although Hammond did not expect this board merely to carry out his opinions, he did not hesitate to express his views on possible changes to its chairman (Satterlee). The new surgeon general was a "regular" in the medical profession, but at the same time he was restless, imaginative, with a zest for experiment that made him willing to break with tradition if he could advance the health of the troops.[26] The members of the board barely received their appointments when Hammond dictated a letter to Satterlee in which his amanuensis wrote:

> He [Hammond] thinks there should be supplied the Gum Acacia in lump, the Opium also, and the quantity of powdered gum is not sufficient to make the proper quantity of Paregoric and Laudanum. For the former of these official preparations are also needed benzoic acid and anise, neither of which are placed on the Table. A pint of Laudanum is hardly deemed enough for a hospital for six months. Other articles should also be supplied, e.g., acetic extract of colchicum, zinc cerate, the bicarbonate and nitrate of potash, the fluid extract of cubebs or powder, as there are no cubebs at all on the list . . . [27]

The board, after accepting some, but not all of these suggestions, reported on July 15; a new table was then drafted and Hammond promulgated it in a circular on October 20, 1862.[28] This was followed by another revision (announced May 7, 1863) that made relatively few important changes except for the controversial omission of calomel and tartar emetic from the table.[29] After more than two years, largely due to Hammond's influence, the standard supply table had become adequate to the needs of the armies.

A rigid application of the supply table was indicated in the *Revised Regulations* of 1861, which stipulated:

> The medical supplies for the army are prescribed in the standard supply table. When any requisition for medical supplies is not according to the supply table, the reason therefore must be set forth.[30]

This regulation, however, created something of a problem when surgeons, many of whom left the practice of medicine to serve the volunteer regiments of their states, began to treat the sick and wounded. For although the supply table remained firmly in control of the "regulars," there had been a marked increase in the demand for indigenous materia medica in the years that preceded the war. As Procter indicated, there was in progress during that era "a voluminous mixture of regular medicine, and new discoveries in the literature of Eclecticism." While the "regulars" of the army's Medical Department might stand by their "mineral medications," there were those in the ranks of the volunteer army who rejoiced that numerous indigenous plants were finding their way into the United States Pharmacopoeia.[31] Surgeons might therefore be expected to diverge from the standard supply table, with or without authorization from a superior, to test their therapeutic convictions. In the West, William R. Smith Jr. treated camp dysentery with "extraordinary success" at a Cairo, Illinois, post hospital by combining a fluid ounce of fluidextract of redbud *(Cercis canadensis)* with three fluid ounces of aromatic syrup of rhubarb.[32] In another illustration drawn from a different theater of the war after Gettysburg, we find a volunteer assistant receiving permission from the hard-pressed surgeons of the V Corps to pour coal oil into suppurating wounds.[33] Many another country doctor, well versed in his herbals and eclectic formulas, became a problem for Charles S. Tripler, the medical director of the Army of the Potomac in 1861. He summarized his dilemma and explained his solution when he said:

> The volunteer medical officers being many of them country doctors accustomed to a village nostrum practice, could not readily change their habits and accustom themselves to the rigid system of the army in regard to their supplies. To meet the difficulty I attempted within reasonable limits to disregard supply tables, and to give the surgeons articles of medicine and hospital stores to suit even their caprices, if in my

judgment such articles could be of any avail in the treatment of disease . . . [34]

The medical purveyor of the army, however, was not so liberal in his interpretation of the regulations. He insisted upon submitting all extraordinary requisitions to Surgeon General Finley, who would not permit anything that was not on the supply table to be issued without his personal consent.[35] Tripler's orders not only were countermanded, but he found that when he himself wished to prescribe whiskey and quinine as a prophylactic against malarial fevers, it was necessary to ask the United States Sanitary Commission to give him a small amount of the drug for his experiment. After he received favorable reports on its effectiveness, the surgeon general gave him permission to issue it in "reasonable quantities" to the regiments.[36] It soon became well established.

When Hammond followed the ultraconservative Finley in the surgeon general's office, he informed Jonathan Letterman, Tripler's successor as medical director of the Army of the Potomac, that he was no stickler who followed the letter of the supply table. He instructed Letterman, "You are authorized to call directly upon the Medical Purveyors in Washington, Baltimore, Philadelphia and New York, who will be directed to furnish you everything you ask for, regardless of supply-tables or forms."[37]

The purveyors at the principal depots played a double role in the Medical Department's supply system. They not only issued medical supplies, but they purchased them in the market. Early in the war the authority to procure supplies devolved upon them more or less by implication, there being no other bonded or commissioned officers appointed for that purpose.[38] But an Act of Congress (approved April 6, 1862) directed specifically that "medical purveyors . . . [should] be charged, under the direction of the Surgeon General, with the selection and purchase of all medical supplies."[39] Among the purveyors, those in New York

City (Richard S. Satterlee) and Philadelphia (George E. Cooper) were significant figures.

For many years before the outbreak of the Civil War, the medical and hospital supplies of the United States Army came almost exclusively from the medical purveying depot in New York City. From there they went to subdepots in the south and west—New Orleans, San Antonio, Camp Floyd (Utah), and Albuquerque—for distribution to the army posts. When the war made necessary the expansion of the supply system in 1861, New York City and Philadelphia became even greater supply centers. From them the medicines, surgical instruments, hospital beds, and scores of additional items flowed to other major purveying depots, at Washington, D.C., St. Louis, Cairo (Illinois), Baltimore, Hilton Head, Fortress Monroe, Newbern, New Orleans, Memphis, Nashville, Louisville, Chicago, and still others near large bodies of troops and convenient to land or water transportation routes. Before the war ended, a maximum of thirty depots were in operation.[40] The medical purveyors at the various depots, in addition to drawing supplies for their warehouses from the principal purveying depots in New York City and Philadelphia, made direct purchases in other cities, such as Baltimore, Louisville, St. Louis, and Washington, D.C.[41]

Establishing the purveying depots at widely scattered points also called for responsible persons who would be familiar with the drugs to superintend the sorting, storage, and forwarding of the medical supplies from the depots to purveying officers in the field or hospitals. Such positions seemed to offer an opportunity to pharmacists. In January 1862, the editor of the *American Journal of Pharmacy* suggested that pharmacists serving with the United States Army should be given "a distinct standing and the rank of pharmaceutist as in the French army."[42] The surgeons of the Medical Department, who reflected the traditionally critical attitude of the medical profession toward pharmaceutical "handmaidens,"[43] took no notice of such proposals, but in an offhand way a few skilled pharmacists received an opportunity to serve when, on May 20, 1862, Congress authorized the secretary of war to appoint six medical storekeepers. One clause in the measure required that they should be "skilled apothecaries or druggists" between twenty-five and forty years of age. Those who qualified for these positions were required to pass an examination in "the ordinary branches of a good English education," pharmacy, and materia medica. They had no rank, but by courtesy they were usually addressed as "Captain," and after posting a $40,000 bond, they received, issued, and were held accountable for the medical stores in the purveying depots' warehouses; four of the six also served concurrently as acting medical purveyors with the authority to purchase medical supplies.[44] Hammond had words of praise for this "most useful class of officers," and expressed regret that the statute, which created the positions, had authorized too small a number.[45] No further appointments were made, however, and at the end of the war only five of them were still on active duty.[46]

Not all the medicines received by soldiers in the Union armies came through the medical purveying depots. The regiments of volunteers at times not only received their arms and uniforms from their state governments, but medical supplies as well. Frederick Stearns, a prominent member of the pharmaceutical profession in Detroit, served as medical purveyor to the Michigan troops. He expanded his small shop with an attached laboratory into a pharmaceutical manufacturing establishment that required a four-story building.[47] The subsistence department of the United States Army procured some drugs early in the war.[48] Under army regulations, when a medical disbursing officer could not be reached, the officers in the Quartermaster Department might purchase medical supplies by filling out an appropriate form. This practice led to difficulties when the Medical Department was forced to rely on the Quartermaster Department, particularly in transporting drugs.[49] A case in point, five days after the battle of

Gettysburg, Medical Inspector Edward P. Vollum arrived at the scene of the battle to find the demand for disinfectants, iodine, tincture of iron and other drugs so urgent that he purchased some of them in the town, and sent the bills to the quartermaster there for payment.[50]

At Mower General Hospital, located on a small plateau near the village of Chestnut Hill, about nine miles from Philadelphia, hospital stewards operated their own small manufacturing laboratory in a stone building $(14' \times 16')$ ventilated only by an open skylight (see Photo 1.1). With a "large-sized cooking stove, and some of the more ordinary apparatus," which did not include a percolator, they prepared tinctures in quantities varying from one-half gallon to ten gallons, and also fluid extracts. Even though they lacked the "proper means for the nice regulation of heat used in evaporating," a few solid extracts, together with "most of the syrups, cerates, ointments, wines and waters of the Pharmacopoeia" were likewise produced, none in sufficient quantity, however, to supply the hospital's needs. As did other general hospitals, Mower relied mainly upon drugs that came to it through the purveying depots.[51]

There were, of course, many "boys in blue" who refused to report their illnesses, preferring to treat their own afflictions with homespun remedies, or patronizing vendors of proprietary drugs who often directed their advertising toward the armies. The makers of T. M. Sharp's Pills—"Positive Cure For Dyspepsia"—reproduced in their lithograph a testimonial from a satisfied user of their preparation in the Second Minnesota Volunteers, who wrote: "I have used a few Boxes of your excellent Pills, and I now send money for two boxes. . . . The Army doctors are not the best in the world."[52] Another lithographed poster presented an anachronistic biblical tableau, with Moses handing out Holloway's Pills and Ointments to soldiers, civilians, and freed slaves.[53] At times the ubiquitous sutlers peddled citrate of magnesia, bicarbonate of soda, citric and tartaric acid, and cream of

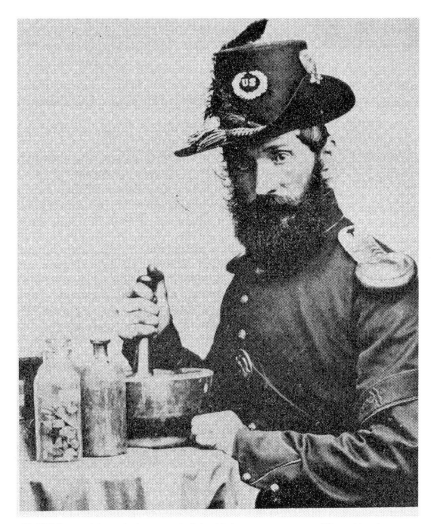

PHOTO 1.1. A hospital steward of the Union army poses stiffly at his pharmaceutical duties.

tartar to the officers and soldiers of the Army of the Cumberland.[54] C. L. Barton & Co., a firm that prepared "Dr. Velloc's Pink Cerate" with a claim that it would exterminate lice and itch, established a depot for its manufacture in Nashville (after the federal occupation of that city) and another in Washington, D.C.[55] Even President Lincoln urged Hammond to permit a trial of one of Dr. Forsha's medicines for the treatment of gunshot wounds. After testing it, Hammond denounced this concoction as "a very irritating and pungent preparation" that had the odor of cedar oil and aggravated the sufferings of several wounded officers to whom Forsha administered it after the battle of Cedar Mountain.[56]

Bizarre attempts to circumvent the services of the Medical Department notwithstanding, the great bulk of medical supplies reached the army through the regular medical purveying channels. From the purveying depots nearest to the major engagements, the medicines were issued to the field purveyor, who supplied the men in the field by keeping up with the troops. When, for example, the Army of the Potomac moved to the Rappahannock River in November 1862, that army's purveyor shifted his field depot from Harper's Ferry to Washington, D.C., and then to Aquia Creek, where his drugs were made accessible to the corps in camp at Falmouth by a short railroad.[57] From his advance depot, usually as close as possible to the fighting, the field purveyor or his assistants (usually hospital stewards) refilled the medicine wagon attached to each brigade. If he was otherwise unoccupied, the army purveyor (who was also a United States Army surgeon) gave emergency treatment to the wounded and even performed surgery.[58]

Experimentation was begun in 1862 with a light, mobile medicine wagon that could travel with the ambulances and still carry sufficient drugs and other supplies for field duty. E. Hayes & Co. of Wheeling constructed such a vehicle from plans and specifications provided by Jonathan Letterman, medical director of the Army of the Potomac. Later in the same year, Jacob Dunton of Philadelphia, a businessman, presented another design, which was rejected. T. Morris Perot, a businessman of the same city, met the requirements, however, with a wagon that came to be identified with his name. The cost of furnishing it with supplies was high, but "the fixtures and arrangements for transporting supplies in this wagon were excellent and convenient." It was finally superseded by the famous Autenrieth wagon, which was adopted upon recommendation of an army medical board in June 1864. Further improvements on this design were made in turn upon wagons constructed at government shops before the end of the war.[59]

The Medical Department apparently considered the improved medicine wagons to be one of its great achievements.[60] In the autumn of 1865, Surgeon General Barnes instructed the medical purveyor at Philadelphia to construct a medicine wagon (with labels substituted for perishable drugs in its contents) for the Industrial Exhibition to be held in Paris.[61] A considerable number of these wagons were stored in St. Louis, instead of being sold as surplus at the end of the war, and were held there for issue to the army on the western frontier.[62]

Second only to the medicine wagons in importance for distributing supplies to men in the field, were the medical panniers. Early in the war these were wooden, similar to the medicine chests used by country doctors, on sailing ships, and by provincial militia troops as far back as the colonial era.[63] Large, heavy chests continued to be carried in common army wagons throughout the war, but only to provide reserve medical supplies for refilling knapsacks and panniers. By 1863, the panniers began to be made in new designs, which were conceived by Edward R. Squibb and others. Squibb's pannier had an iron frame covered with cowhide, the hair left on the skin and turned outward; it could be either lashed to a packsaddle or hung from a saddle on one side of a horse or mule if counterbalanced by an equal weight.[64] Each regiment was allowed one mule to carry its field panniers.[65] Even though the new panniers were lighter than the wooden chests, they were still inconveniently borne by the animals and instead generally were found under the front seats of the ambulance wagons.[66]

The iron-framed panniers were about the same size as the wooden medicine chests which Hammond decreed they should succeed (21 inches long, 11½ inches wide, and 11⅜ inches deep). Forty-nine pharmaceuticals packed in tin bottles and lacquer-coated boxes were fitted into the two compartments of each pannier, with additional space for extracts of coffee and beef, condensed milk,[67] black tea, sugar, and emergency surgical instruments—cupping tins, probangs, scissors, syringes, tourniquets, and sponges. There were also adhesive plaster, lint, matches, oiled silk, roller bandages, tape, note paper, pens, candles, graduated measures, scales and weights, spatulas, and another score of items.[68] Unlike most of the drugs purchased by the federal government, those found in these panniers were supplied by Squibb and others such as Jacob Dunton of Philadelphia, under contracts with the Medical Department, for $111 each if purchased on credit (as many of them were), or for cash at slightly less. (Squibb was ready to produce them for $100.93 cash in the spring of 1863.)[69]

Each medical officer in the field also received one medical knapsack, which weighed between eighteen and twenty pounds. At first made of light wood, they were later of "wicker-work, covered with canvas or enamelled cloth"; and finally there was a still lighter case of leather, the "field companion," which the medical officer could suspend on a strap over his shoulder. Such cases did not entirely supersede knapsacks, however, carried by orderlies or hospital stewards, who accompanied the surgeons to the battlefields.[70]

The hospital stewards were indeed a most able class of personnel. In addition to following the armies closely into battle with knapsacks on their backs, as the constant assistants of the surgeons, they skillfully performed many tasks in the hospitals: they supervised the cooks and nurses, kept medical records and accounts, and in emergencies when the surgeons were absent they performed minor surgical operations and prescribed medicines.[71] For their instruction, Joseph Janvier Woodward, an assistant surgeon in the surgeon general's office, prepared a *Hospital Steward's Manual,* which, among other topics, gave elementary instructions for managing a dispensary and a few hints on pharmacy.[72]

A general order signed on February 2, 1859, stipulated that hospital stewards who were enlisted men, not commissioned officers, were to be "sufficiently intelligent and skilled in pharmacy for the discharge of responsible duties. . . ."[73] In 1861, one hospital steward was allowed to each company of troops in the field, and one to each army post.[74] The next year, a statute authorized as many as the surgeon general thought necessary;[75] but by August, there were only 200 of them in service.[76] Letterman, however, directed that they should be attached to every field hospital.[77]

If no steward was present, the commanding officer might assign an enlisted man to perform the duties upon recommendation of a medical officer in his command, and if the soldier carried out his duties satisfactorily, he might be given such an appointment.[78] Some hospital stewards, therefore, did not begin as pharmacists, but rather acquired some knowledge of pharmaceutical skills while in the army. One of these stewards, Charles Beneulyn Johnson of the 130th Illinois Volunteers, recalled that he had been able to get his position "not because I was well qualified for the place as I should have been, but because I was the best fitted for it of anyone available." Discussing his qualifications, he continued,

I had a little Latin, a little chemistry, a little physics, a little higher mathematics before joining the army, and very shortly after I entered I began familiarizing myself with drugs and chemicals, and with such other duties as might fall to a hospital attache . . . [79]

Many of the young stewards, on the other hand, were pharmacists who left retail shops short-handed professionally, as they decided to apply their skills to the work of the Medical Department.[80] A number of them became distinguished members of their profession and leaders in public life after the war. James Vernor of Detroit, a hospital steward for two years before he received a lieutenant's commission, became a member of Michigan's first Board of Pharmacy after he returned to civilian life, and for a quarter of a century he held a seat on the Detroit City Council.[81] Another brilliant pharmacist, Joseph Lyon Lemberger, left his pharmacy in Lebanon, Pennsylvania (he graduated from the Philadelphia College of Pharmacy in 1854), to serve as a hospital steward; later he helped to organize the Pennsylvania Pharmaceutical Association and was president of the American Pharmaceutical Association (1905-1906).[82] Another able Pennsylvanian, George W. Kennedy, who wrote more than fifty articles for the leading journals of his profession while he operated a pharmacy in Pottsville, enlisted in a Pennsylvania Reserve Regiment. He was wounded and sent to an army general hospital in Philadelphia; during his convalescence he attended lectures at the Philadelphia College of Pharmacy, then reenlisted and served the last two years of the war as a hospital steward.[83] There were rewards and experiences in pharmacy at war that must have been entirely disproportionate to a steward's $30 monthly salary.

The personnel of the field purveying system received definite quantities of medical supplies for distribution: one knapsack to each regimental medical officer, a medicine chest or pannier to each regiment, and one hospital wagon to each brigade. When filled, these were supposed to provide enough medical supplies for one month's service in the field.[84] One common army wagon also carried medical and hospital supplies for each regiment in the supply train. Each division hospital had its own supplies, hauled in three army wagons and one medical wagon.[85] In 1862, Jonathan Letterman, medical director of the Army of the Potomac, instituted a supply table for that army with definite allowances of drugs to be issued by the field purveyor to the brigade surgeons, who in turn were to dole them out to the regiments.[86] This table, containing a selected list of drugs from the standard supply table, was periodically revised, and continued in effect until the end of the war.[87]

In spite of the reforms brought about by Letterman and others in the distribution of medical supplies, bitter criticisms of the system were not infrequent. Early in the war, higher medical officers and surgeons in the field chronically underestimated the amounts of supplies required in the field and hospital. The problem of logistics was ever present, especially because of the Quartermaster Department's inability to get the drugs to the places where they were most needed at a given time. In Hammond's words, "Much suffering . . . [was] caused by the impossibility of furnishing supplies to the wounded, when those supplies were [with]in a few miles in great abundance."[88] Surgeon Charles S. Tripler declared that medical officers in the Army of the Potomac had to go into Washington, D.C., for medicines and deliver them to the camps.[89] Hammond finally induced the War Department to set up a Bureau of Medical Transportation in the surgeon general's office.

The shortcomings were not entirely those of the Quartermaster Department. The lack of moveable depots and field hospitals impeded the flow of supplies from the central depots to the field. The practice of supplying medical stores to each regiment led to competition among them, which resulted in an excess of medicines for some while others went without.[90] There was wastefulness. For example, after the peninsular campaign of 1862, McClellan's army was evacuated, and left behind most of its medical supplies.[91]

Tactical considerations also at times interfered with the medical purveying system in the field. This was true at Gettysburg, where

Meade held the trains far in the rear during the fighting,[92] and at Chickamauga, where Rosecrans' army so far outran its supplies that the medical officers had to rely upon the articles that they carried in their knapsacks.[93]

In the hospitals also, there were complaints about the inefficiency of the purveying system. One volunteer wrote: "We need beds and bedding, hospital clothing and sick-diet, proper medicines, surgical instruments and good nurses. . . . I suppose we shall have them when the government can get around to it, and in the meantime we try to be patient."[94] No matter what the specific causes for grievances, the medical purveying system generally received more than its share of abuse.

Behind the immediate causes for complaint in field purveying, there were major problems involving procurement policies of the Medical Department's purveying system as a whole. These were in one way or another related to the government's dealings with the pharmaceutical industry. When, for example, a therapeutic agent grew rapidly in favor, as did potassium permanganate for the treatment of hospital gangrene, it was sometimes forwarded irregularly or in short supply because of unperfected processes or production resources of the manufacturing chemists who were producing it.[95] The medical purveyors, moreover, through bargaining with private dealers for drugs and chemicals, became deeply involved in the drug market. During the first half of the war a large proportion of the medical supplies (in June 1863, nine-tenths of them) were procured in the open market.[96]

From the government's standpoint the market conditions were anything but satisfactory. Imported crude drugs were frequently in either short or irregular supply. Cream of tartar had been a favorite with speculators for two years before the war. During the secession crisis, cubebs were held at extreme rates; vanilla beans were priced almost out of the market; and there was a speculative surge in the demand for licorice paste, cardamom, balsam of copaiba, tolu, cumin seed, senna, saffron, asafetida, nutgalls, jalap, and rhubarb. The essential oils and lime and lemon juices from Sicily were imported erratically, and even in 1860 there was a reduced stock of cinchona bark on both the American and British markets.[97] Formosa camphor was a closely guarded monopoly controlled by the Taotai of the island.[98] The supply of bismuth from the mines of Saxony and Bohemia was at least temporarily unequal to an increased demand for the metal in Europe and the United States.[99]

As the dollar fell in value during the war, in relation to European currencies, the exchange rate climbed rapidly, with scarce and high-priced drugs, such as opium, quickly reflecting the fluctuations. The cost of drugs responded to the rise and fall of gold more than most other commodities.[100] Prices of imported drugs were also swept upward by the interruption of direct trade between the United States and distant ports of Asia and Africa, caused by the raids (actual or anticipated) of the Confederate commerce destroyers, by the strained diplomatic relations with Great Britain and France, and by the monopolistic controls exercised by a few importing houses.[101] Although the federal government could purchase in bond the imported drugs which it needed, thus escaping tariff duties,[102] Congress increased the tariff rates during each wartime session, and drug prices often rose in anticipation of these changes. "The drug and spice men," it was said, were always the first to become excited at such times, and the price of domestic and imported drugs usually responded to the stimulus.[103] Shortages in the English drug market were often reflected in American sales. This was especially significant because many articles which before the war had come directly from Asiatic ports were being received from England at higher prices.[104]

Conditions in the domestic drug market created problems for the government even more serious than those related to imported drugs. Early in 1861, anticipating the coming demand for medicines, speculators began to buy up quantities of pharmaceuticals.[105] American manufacturers did little to expand their production of some products. Repeatedly, they raised their price quotations.[106] As Maisch pointed out, some articles on the standard supply table did not join in this advance, and the rise in the price of others did little more than reflect the premium on gold and the higher foreign exchange rate;[107] but some of the leading pharmaceuticals shot upward until a number of them were 500 percent higher by 1863.[108] The Medical Department also found that at times it was necessary for its medical purveyors to pay more than the market quotations. The most closely held drugs were not even quoted in market reports. Transactions involving them, if they were noticed at all, were listed as being carried out on "private terms," or "on terms kept quiet."[109] The supply of indigenous botanicals was often concealed by the dealers.[110]

Most of the market transactions were controlled by drug brokers, whose numbers increased rapidly during the years just before the war. Through handling and subdividing the drug manufacturers' output and the imports, and supplying them to jobbers and retailers, they had won a significant position in the drug trade.[111] Drug exchanges, similar to the petroleum exchange and other organized commodity markets, appeared in both New York City and Philadelphia.[112] "Corners" were evident in a number of the scarce drugs, along with short-selling, "options and puts," and similar operations.[113] One assistant surgeon, after becoming familiar with the New York City drug market, wrote to the medical purveyor in that city: "The drug trade work together as do gold brokers."[114]

The rapidly increasing prices of "articles of need" seriously embarrassed the surgeon general's office.[115] In purchasing scarce drugs, especially quinine sulfate, the medical purveyors turned and twisted to grasp whatever opportunities came their way as they were carried along in the currents of trade. Through telegrams between the surgeon general's office and the New York City purveyor, Hammond (perhaps contrary to the letter of the purveying law of 1862) directed these purchasing operations,

authorizing and then withholding permission to make transactions for small lots (3,000 to 5,000 ounces) of quinine, as the
quotations rose and fell from day to day.[116] The supply of this
most sought after drug was at times dangerously deficient. On
March 20, 1863, as an example, there remained only 2,000 ounces
unappropriated in the New York City purveying depot.[117]

Doubts concerning the government's ability to make payment
possibly caused some to hesitate or even to refuse to sell to the
Medical Department.[118] Those firms which did deal with the
medical purveyors often had to wait, with embarrassment to their
finances, before receiving their money.[119] Instead of cash they
might be given the government's certificates of indebtedness
which could be sold only at a discount on the New York City
money market. On one occasion in 1862, the Medical Department was so completely out of funds that it could not meet its
obligations to a broker who had advanced the money to purchase
on its account 500 ounces of quinine. The New York City purveyor received instructions to promise interest to the broker on
the sum advanced, together with a further promise that the government would pay "enough more than the present worth" of the
drug when it "came into funds."[120]

To free the Medical Department from dependence upon the
vagaries of the market and the drug brokers, the medical purveyors
concentrated their purchases of pharmaceuticals among a few
manufacturers in various cities.[121] In New York City, Satterlee
relied upon the probity of Philip Schieffelin & Co. and Edward R.
Squibb in preference to others who might outbid them in price but
not in the quality of their products. "The Government," Satterlee
explained, "always starts with the quality of the article as the first
consideration, the next is price." In doing this, Satterlee was carrying out a policy fully sanctioned by the surgeon general's office,
especially during the tenure of Hammond, and authenticated by
long-established practice in the army, whose purchasing agents
had exempted medical supplies and gunpowder from competitive

bidding.[122] One Philadelphia manufacturer, John Wyeth and Brother, received most of the government's orders for medical supplies in that city until 1863,[123] although its owner, John Wyeth, purchased some of the more specialized articles from other manufacturers—Henry Bower, Powers & Weightman, and others—to fill the orders,[124] as did Squibb in New York City.

Such practices did not, as Hammond's enemies contended, necessarily indicate either misdemeanors by the surgeon general or dishonesty in the medical purveyors.[125] Rather, they were an attempt to get medicines of acceptable quality for the armies at a time when adulterated products were common[126] and before the development of effective tests for the more complex preparations.[127] In view of the unfavorable conditions under which the government was forced to purchase in the open market, it might also be expected that the government would be relying on certain companies to get a greater variety of supplies more quickly than by purchasing them in small lots from numerous dealers who offered articles of uneven quality.[128]

Hammond also enthusiastically developed a policy of stock-piling medical supplies at the major depots. On July 31, 1862, for example, he sent to George F. Cooper, a medical purveyor in Philadelphia, a controversial order that instructed Cooper to fill up his storehouses with sufficient supplies to serve 100,000 men for six months.[129] Hammond's motives were later impugned by Cooper and others, but his objectives were doubtless to insure the army against shortages during periods of critical need, to provide an even flow of pharmaceuticals from the central depots to the field, and to protect the government against future price rises and fluctuations in the drug market.[130] The large warehouses generally remained filled with supplies until the end of the war.[131]

Such measures, however, left the problems of the purveying system far from a solution. In purchasing for quality rather than from considerations of price, the costs were high. As the Squibb price lists of the period indicate, Squibb's quotations were often above those of other manufacturers.[132] Although Hammond seemed to have complete confidence in the probity of the Wyeth firm, George E. Cooper and others soon accused them of providing the Medical Department with inferior medical supplies.[133] There was evident need for some kind of testing laboratory to check the purity of those wines, liquors, crude drugs, and preparations that could be subjected to simple chemical and physical testing procedures, thus assuring more uniform quality of the government's pharmaceuticals.[134] In short, if the Medical Department needed the drug market brokers and pharmaceutical manufacturers, it also needed a more effective yardstick to measure their activities and to strengthen the government's position in its dealings with them. In addition, the Medical Department thought it could reduce costs by manufacturing and processing at least a portion of its own pharmaceutical preparations. By the fall of 1862, Hammond decided that the creation of United States Army Laboratories to test and to manufacture medical supplies for the army was the best answer to his question.

Various explanations for the establishment of the United States Army Laboratories have been given, but W. C. Spencer, in an official report describing the operations of the medical purveying system, probably has stated them most succinctly as follows:

> The quantity and cost of the medicines, hospital stores, dressings, bedding and clothing required for the use of the troops had at this time become so great that the advisability of their preparation and manufacture by the department itself came under consideration. The advantages anticipated from the measure were: — the ability to ascertain in every instance the purity of the wines, liquors, hospital stores and crude drugs offered to the department; the attainment of perfect purity and reliability in the medicines prepared; the securing of uniformity in the mode of putting up supplies for issue and the saving to the Government of a great part of the profit made by ordinary dealers.[135]

Hammond's successor as surgeon general, Joseph K. Barnes, similarly described the advantages of such laboratories as

> . . . perfect purity of drugs, reduction of cost to the full amount of manufacturers' profits which vary from 12 to 33 per cent, uniformity of preparation, the packages having an established form and U.S. Mark . . . and the facilities for correct analysis of all articles liable to adulteration previous to purchase.[136]

A precedent existed. In 1852, the United States Navy had successfully established a manufacturing laboratory in a building originally constructed as a pest house at the United States Naval Hospital in Brooklyn. At the suggestion of C. O. Whelan, supervisor of the hospital, Benjamin F. Bache became director of the laboratory, ably assisted by Edward R. Squibb. When Squibb resigned his post in 1857, the laboratory was manufacturing drugs of the "highest quality" at costs "not greater" than the navy had formerly paid for "inferior" medicines. It was while he was at this laboratory that Squibb developed his steam process for ether, perfected his chloroform-making apparatus, and began to make fluid extracts by what he called repercolation. Bache and Squibb also performed assays and set acceptable standards not only for the drugs they tested, but for other supplies procured by contract—dyes, clothing, blankets, candles, soap, whiskey, and vinegar.[137]

Surgeon General Hammond specifically called attention to the United States Naval Laboratory in proposing similar laboratories for the army.[138] There is no doubt that Hammond originated the army laboratory idea. According to one of his closest associates in the surgeon general's office, Hammond "early and frequently expressed his belief that the Government could manufacture its medicines more economically than it could buy them."[139] If it could not avoid the high price of crude drugs, the Medical Department could at least purchase them in bulk, then subdivide and process them for use in the field and hospitals.[140]

Hammond probably conceived the idea of government laboratories for the manufacture of the army's pharmaceuticals without requiring any suggestions from others. But about the same time that he was formulating his plans, his incoming mail brought proposals that advocated such establishments. E. H. Moore of Dubuque, Iowa, a pharmacist of ten years' experience, wrote one such letter to Secretary of War Stanton, who forwarded it to Hammond. Moore argued that the government's savings would be immense if it could free itself from dependency on the drug manufacturers. He continued:

> I understand that the government is dependent entirely upon the manufacturers for everything used in the way of medicine. While it is necessary to buy chemicals of them, it seems to me that it would be an immense saving to the government if they had a department at Washington, where their Tinctures, Ointments & Syrups might be made & where everything used in the medical department should be sent & there put up in right sized packages & shipped to different purveyors.

Moore professed to foresee no reason why the government's manufacture of drugs should not extend into the postwar era. Perhaps needless to say, he also offered his services as supervisor of the proposed laboratory.[141]

Hammond refused to give him any encouragement, but a similar proposal from one of the medical storekeepers, Hennell Stevens, a former manufacturer of drugs in Philadelphia and a graduate of the Philadelphia College of Pharmacy, secured from the surgeon general a request that Stevens should draft a plan for such an establishment. The result was that Stevens' "Plan for the Establishment of a Purchasing and Manufacturing Depot for the Medical Department of the Army," a handwritten document of about fourteen pages, reached the surgeon general's office about the time that Hammond was beginning his own laboratory project.[142] It probably had little effect upon the planning, but Hammond nevertheless referred it to his medical purveyor in New York City, Richard S. Satterlee, who scornfully replied that Stevens' reasoning was "purely theoretical and fallacious."[143]

Stevens, however, in his first letter to Hammond on the subject, in December, made one suggestion that might well have influenced the surgeon general. This was for the government to lease existing facilities where "hands in government employ" might "put up" tinctures, ointments, and other preparations. "Such an establishment," Stevens wrote, "would involve no expenditure for apparatus and no permanent outlay. At the close of the war if thought advisable, the buildings could be given up, the hands discharged, and the establishment closed."[144] Whatever Hammond may have thought of Stevens' suggestions, Stevens' flashy pretensions as a drug manufacturer in Philadelphia during the 1850s, without actually establishing himself there as one of the substantial manufacturers, apparently influenced Hammond against entrusting him with the supervision of a government laboratory. Stevens remained a medical storekeeper throughout the war.[145]

It was another medical storekeeper, Robert T. Creamer, who was the first to induce Hammond to put into operation a limited experiment in the preparation of pharmaceuticals. A self-styled "practical druggist"[146] from New Jersey who became a medical storekeeper on August 13, 1862,[147] Creamer also became acting medical purveyor in St. Louis in the autumn of 1862 because of the absence of the regular medical purveyor from that city. Near the end of October, Creamer began his maneuvering in a letter addressed to Surgeon General Hammond in which he complained that the medical supplies at the St. Louis purveying depot were insufficient.[148] Although he soon changed his attitude about the quantitative inadequacy of the medical supplies, admitting in December that there was in St. Louis "a large surplus of many supplies," Creamer next requested that such pharmaceuticals as sweet spirit of nitre, Syrup of Squill, and Camphorated Tincture of Opium should be sent to him in bulk rather than in small packages.[149] By quoting items from the J. H. Reed and Company price list, he demonstrated that the Reed firm was selling bottled and packaged drugs to the government at large markups, and glibly added that he could save the Medical Department considerable sums each year "by putting up my own supplies on the premises, in the requisite form in accordance with the 'Supply Table.'" If this were done, empty bottles and vials then "wasted or sold in the Hospitals for trifling value" could be washed and refilled in his "workshop," which would be staffed with "lads and girls at comparatively cheap labor."[150]

Hammond was sufficiently receptive to Creamer's proposals, especially at the prospect of saving through the repeated use of bottles, to authorize the St. Louis storekeeper to carry out his suggestions for putting up drugs "as far as you can do so."[151] But Hammond was so little impressed with Creamer's workshop that he either forgot about it or forgot that he had authorized Creamer to manufacture drugs there. For over two months afterward, he inquired of the assistant surgeon general about what "laboratory" Creamer was referring to in his correspondence with the surgeon general's office.[152]

Creamer, however, had no doubts about his authority. He announced that most of the materia medica in the St. Louis depot's requisitions would be supplied "by the Laboratory now attached to this depot."[153] Between March 1 and July 31, 1863, no less than seventy-eight articles on the standard supply table were issued from the "work room." Most of them were only bottled or packaged there; but others, including Cantharidis Ceratum, a number of fluid extracts, opium pills, and Syrup of Squill were, according to Creamer's reports, manufactured there. The quantities were almost always small: 2,412 ounces of catechu (258 cans); 1,792 ounces of sulfate of cinchona (117 cans); 2,116 ounces of camphor (169 cans); 10,714 ounces of tincture of opium (998 bottles); and

1,664 pounds of Syrup of Squill, to indicate a few of the representative articles.[154]

Creamer's undoing came about as the result of authority to purchase the raw materials processed in his laboratory. Whiskey and wine were two of these products that soon brought forth angry protests of their unfitness for human consumption. The officials at the Memphis purveying depot were especially vehement in condemning the wine that Creamer bottled at St. Louis. The result was that on July 25, the surgeon general "in consequence of reports of the bad quality of articles furnished at your depot," ordered that Creamer should make no more purchases of medical supplies.[155] The laboratory operations were permitted to continue, but Creamer was told that the articles that he put up were "only to meet ordinary demands and for the present."[156] After further exposures of inferior whiskey traced to Creamer's purchases and other complaints against his workshop, including one that his filled bottles were short in weight, the surgeon general ordered Creamer to liquidate the indebtedness of the St. Louis purveying depot and to requisition all his supplies from the medical purveyor in Louisville. Creamer's workshop activities then apparently ground to a halt.[157]

If the St. Louis experiment was a failure, it also demonstrated Hammond's dissatisfaction with the procurement system then in force. Long before Creamer was ordered to curtail his workshop, Hammond was ready to attempt a more comprehensive and effective plan for improving the purveying system through government laboratories. Using the United States Naval Laboratory as an example, he proposed in his annual report (dated November 10, 1862) to the secretary of war that he should be given the authority to establish "a laboratory from which the medical department could draw its supplies of chemical and pharmaceutical preparations." It would be, he declared, "a measure of great utility and economy."[158]

Chapter 2

The Beginnings
of the Laboratories

Surgeon General William A. Hammond was mercurial, imaginative, and impatient with bureaucratic delays. It was typical of him not to wait for slow-moving Congress to act on his request for permission to establish United States Army pharmaceutical laboratories. Instead, he acted. There was not even explicit consent from Secretary of War Stanton, with whom he had quarreled immediately after taking office.[1]

On January 12, 1863, Hammond directed Andrew Kingsbury Smith, then medical director of transportation in Philadelphia, "to seek for a building in or near Philadelphia, suitable for a chemical laboratory for the Med[ical] Dep[artment]." Hammond also directed that the building "should contain room for the preparation of Extracts and Tinctures, and for the subdivision of supplies received in original packages, suitable for Army use."[2] Similar instructions went to Charles McCormick, who had served as Major General Benjamin F. Butler's medical director in New Orleans, to look for a "suitable house for a laboratory" in or near New York City.[3] Hammond arrived at an understanding with Quartermaster General Montgomery C. Meigs, whereby the quartermaster department agreed to rent the laboratories and furnish the necessary fixtures.[4]

McCormick selected a group of three buildings at Astoria, Long Island,* formerly occupied by a manufacturing chemist,

---

*Astoria is in Queens, but at the time Queens County was not yet incorporated into New York City.

John Hyer Jr., which apparently contained some of the more bulky machinery needed for operations; a fourth building was procured nearby in April.[5] With no other authority than Hammond's "verbal permission," McCormick began in January to engage employees for the Astoria laboratory. Hammond then directed the New York medical purveyor, Richard S. Satterlee, to provide the funds necessary to pay their wages.[6]

McCormick had just begun the laboratory project at Astoria when Hammond ordered Andrew K. Smith to visit the United States Naval Laboratory and the Squibb works in Brooklyn, prior to establishing the other laboratory in Philadelphia.[7] At the end of February, Hammond formally requested that Smith be assigned to Robert Murray, medical purveyor at Philadelphia, "for duty in connection with the preparation of medical supplies."[8] On March 9, 1863, Special Order No. 113 (Adjutant General's Office) directed Smith to report to Purveyor Murray, and instructions were sent immediately from Hammond's office to "organize an establishment for the manufacture of drugs."[9]

Smith refused to wait for a formal order from the Adjutant General's Office before beginning to organize his laboratory. In Philadelphia he lost no time in finding, at Sixth and Oxford Streets, a brick establishment owned by Powers & Weightman, but once used by the Crew family's chemical firm.[10] Later, it was a warehouse for pharmaceutical products of John Wyeth and Brother, with quantities of such articles still stored there when the government rented the building.[11] "It is of ample size," Smith advised Hammond, "not only for the preparation of Extracts and tinctures, but for such other pharmaceutical operations as we may gradually take up. . . ."[12] The steam engine, a crushing mill, shafting and belting, and "various other conveniences" were still in place.[13] Smith did not inform Hammond, however, that the premises bore the marks of a flood which had swept through that part of Philadelphia only six months before he wrote his glowing description.[14] Possible objections that Powers & Weightman might present to the government's leasing their building for competing operations he dismissed by explaining, "I will tell them . . . that this will make no difference as we will have a laboratory anyway."[15] He was correct.

Within a fortnight he forwarded an offer from Powers & Weightman to sell or lease the property,[16] and Hammond then asked Meigs to negotiate a ten-year lease agreement.[17] This contract, signed on February 2, 1863, called for rent of $208 per month, and the lease was to run for "not over five years."[18] Since the proposed laboratory was identified by Hammond as "a storehouse for drugs and Medical supplies," the quartermaster department paid the rent for the building, and the surgeon general's office merely agreed to assume that share which could be charged to the machinery used for "the preparation of powders and extracts."[19]

Smith was not content with one structure for his laboratory. Nearby, at Sixth and Master Streets, there was the former carriage factory of W. D. Rogers which the government was renting as a hospital.[20] He quickly informed Hammond: "The hospital can be closed immediately without detriment to the service as there are now 1865 vacant beds in the city and vicinity. . . ."[21] Hammond responded with an order that the hospital be evacuated and turned over to Smith for use as an annex to the laboratory.[22] Smith also visited other temporary hospitals that had been closed as others opened in Philadelphia. After his scavenging tour he reported to Hammond:

> I have gleaned from the hospitals which have been closed everything which will be of advantage to me and in that way have secured gas, steam, & water piping. I have taken one of the upright boilers for an ammonia still, and that will save us $125 at least, & our tables, platform scales & a multitude of useful articles have been secured from the same source . . .[23]

By making "a great many alterations" in the principal laboratory building (Sixth and Oxford Streets) and devoting himself "to the laboratory all day, and [to] dreams about [the] laboratory all night," Smith was able to boast that within a week after his formal appointment his apparatus had been ordered, and indeed by then the tubs, percolators, and vats were arriving daily.[24] On May 1, 1863, the Philadelphia laboratory was ready to deliver medical preparations.[25]

With little planning, Hammond improvised as he created the laboratories, often without leaving any record of his actions. His successor in the surgeon general's office, Joseph K. Barnes, while admitting that it was impossible to unravel Hammond's complicated negotiations, was inclined to believe that Hammond did not go to the secretary of war (Edwin M. Stanton) for any authorization to set up the laboratories.[26] Instead, Hammond avoided a possible refusal from the war office by making the laboratories adjuncts to the New York City and Philadelphia purveying depots, and, consequently, a legitimate expenditure for the Medical and Hospital Department funds.[27] In Barnes' words, Hammond did not seek "either the authority of law or the sanction of the War Office."[28] Nevertheless, Barnes erred if he implied that Hammond acted entirely without the knowledge or implied consent of the War Department. Personnel for the laboratories were transferred by special orders of the adjutant general's staff. The Quartermaster Department leased the laboratory buildings, and finally, on April 20, after the laboratories were becoming a reality, Hammond requisitioned $200,000, payable in certificates of indebtedness. These requisitions were accepted by the secretary of war, and the sums were made available "solely for the payment for apparatus, raw material and the expenses" of the laboratories.[29]

The expedient decision to place the laboratories under the jurisdiction of the medical purveyors in Philadelphia and New York City was a cause of friction from the beginning. Each purveyor was responsible for his laboratory's property. He was also "ordered to keep the accounts, disburse monies required,"[30] handle all requisitions of apparatus,[31] purchase the raw drugs, and control the payrolls. All medicines produced in the laboratories were to be issued through the purveyors, and even official correspondence of the laboratory directors was to be routed through the purveying offices. The purveyors were, in effect, responsible to the surgeon general for the laboratory operations.

But in practice, Hammond often bypassed the purveyors to deal directly with the laboratory directors so that although the "ultimate responsibility for the management" of the laboratories remained with the medical purveyor, their active direction was beyond the scope of his activities.[32] Until his visits to New York City and Philadelphia were brusquely curtailed by Stanton, Hammond at times appeared in person to supervise the formative stages of the laboratories' development.[33] Both before and after his travel was limited, Hammond called Smith and McCormick to Washington for conferences "on business connected with the preparation of medical supplies."[34] Hammond's assistant, Joseph Janvier Woodward, on occasion made inspection tours.[35] But it was mainly through informal correspondence between Hammond and Smith that Hammond maintained contact with the Philadelphia laboratory. Hammond, for example, personally approved the appointment of the brilliant pharmacist John M. Maisch as the chief chemist,[36] and even became interested in such details as the design to be placed on the package labels.[37]

There was never such close rapport between the surgeon general's office and McCormick, but Hammond unsuccessfully tried to coordinate the activities of the two laboratories by setting up a two-member board, composed of the two directors, with McCormick as president, to "arrange the plan of operation . . . at New York and Philadelphia . . . so as to secure entire concord of action in all particulars." The instructions continued,

You will adopt such standard labels, bottles, boxes, cans and other packages as may seem to you best, and arrange a uniform system of packing. You will also specify what articles of the supply table can be manufactured to advantage, what powdered, purified and otherwise prepared for issue from the raw material.[38]

McCormick and Smith met as a board and agreed upon labels that would be similar although not identical for the two laboratories, but they found little business to transact and Smith complained that they were embarrassed "by non-receipt of instructions for its [the board's] government."[39] When McCormick left the Astoria laboratory soon after that, the board was not reconstituted.

In contrast to Hammond's success in putting the Philadelphia laboratory into operation, Astoria made slow progress in the spring of 1863. Various causes were responsible for this lag, but foremost was the obstructive attitude of Satterlee, abetted by Edward Robinson Squibb. When Squibb heard of the projected laboratory, he remarked, "Othello's occupation is (nearly) gone."[40]

Satterlee's role was quite different from that of the medical purveyor in Philadelphia, Robert Murray, who replaced George E. Cooper in October, 1862.[41] Murray, in his early forties, was young for a medical purveyor or even for an army surgeon. Until he was appointed medical director of transportation in Philadelphia a short time before he became purveyor, his wartime experience had been in the western theater of the war. After the battle of Perryville, he had become medical director of the 14th Army Corps and the Department of the Cumberland.[42] Early in 1863, when Hammond and Smith were organizing the Philadelphia laboratory, Murray did not seem to resent possible encroachment upon his authority. Later in the war, when he mentioned that his control over laboratory policies was more nominal than real,[43] there were indications of increased tension between him and

Smith, but he cooperated in the laboratory project. In fact, John M. Maisch praised Murray warmly for his "zealous aid" that made possible their successful operations.[44] Murray's attitude was almost exactly the reverse of Satterlee's.

In dealing with Satterlee, Hammond was contending with a rock-ribbed conservative of the Army Medical Department, one who was born in the eighteenth century and who received his appointment as assistant surgeon in February 1822. Satterlee served at various posts along the lake frontier, and received a citation for his part in the Battle of Lake Okeechobee during the Seminole War (honorable mention being made in the report of Colonel Zachary Taylor). As a medical officer, he was with the troops that escorted the Cherokee Indians beyond the Mississippi River, and later he was chief surgeon of General Worth's division with Scott's army in Mexico, where he was several times "honorably mentioned for his untiring energy, ability and zealous attachment to duty." After the fall of Mexico City, Scott named him medical director of his entire army.[45]

It was with memories of a long and sometimes brilliant career that Satterlee, in 1854, became attending surgeon and medical purveyor in New York City.[46] He was not only firmly entrenched in the medical purveyor's office by 1861, but his influence far exceeded that usually enjoyed by a purveyor. He was inflexible in his rectitude, and he was suspicious of anything that might be an unsound innovation. For example, when Hammond tactlessly sent Hennell Stevens' bulky plan for an army manufacturing depot[47] for comment, Satterlee considered Stevens' strictures upon existing purveying practices to be a personal insult. He angrily replied,

> There is much danger in trusting to the judgement, reasoning and deductions of a man who has been thoroughly unsuccessful in his own business for years, and through many changes, and who after an experience of only a few months,

in an entirely new sphere, proposes to radically change everything he meets with to conform to his ideas of proper administrative ability, as separate and distinct from accumulated practical knowledge and experience; and who seems to overlook the fact that amid the difficulties of a gigantic war which has absorbed the energies of wiser heads than his, may not be the time for revolutionary changes . . .[48]

Satterlee directed this blast at Hammond far more than at Stevens. It exemplifies the incompatibility that hindered cooperation between the Surgeon General and his New York purveyor in spite of Hammond's attempts to win Satterlee over by such flattery as giving his name to one of the large Philadelphia army hospitals.[49] Satterlee also demonstrated a pique that grew out of the appointment of Hammond over the heads of older aspirants to the surgeon general's office. When Surgeon General Thomas Lawson died (May 1861), the General-in-Chief, Winfield Scott, supported the candidacy of his former medical director, Satterlee; but the promotion went instead to Clement Alexander Finley. He in turn was followed by Hammond (April 25, 1862).[50] If the cold formality of the correspondence between Hammond and Satterlee was a measure of his disappointment, Satterlee never forgave Hammond for taking that most desired prize which he had coveted but lost. Satterlee adopted a petulant tone, reproachfully bidding Hammond to recommend him for promotion to the rank of brigadier general.[51] Possibly to appease his "old and faithful officer," Hammond asked for the promotion[52] (March 1863), but it was September 2, 1864, before Satterlee received his citation as brevet brigadier general,[53] and it was 1866 before he was a full lieutenant colonel in the regular army.

At the outset of the Astoria venture it was Hammond's intention that Satterlee should "regulate the expenditures and operations of the laboratory" according to his own judgment and remain in close touch with it.[54] Satterlee's rejection of this role[55] forced Hammond to ask him the direct question, "What articles [do] you think from your experience may be manufactured at the laboratory profitable to the government?"[56] To this Satterlee replied, "I have the honor to state, that taking into account the expense of the laboratory, viz. building, apparatus, operations, etc., I doubt if we can manufacture anything to advantage. That is, and has been . . . my opinion . . ."[57] Hammond then lost patience and brought the issue to a climax:

> The Surgeon General is loth to believe that manufacturing chemists and druggists generally are so superior in skill and business qualifications to yourself and the other med. officers who may be placed in charge of the laboratory, that our efforts alone should be prosecuted to disadvantage while theirs are attended with success. The Surgeon General regrets that your opinion on the subject differs from his, and desires nevertheless your cordial cooperation, that the business may be conducted, if without advantage still to as little disadvantage as possible.[58]

Satterlee retreated,[59] but he remained unconvinced, and continued as before to raise practical objections to the laboratory's operations. He pointed out, for example, that McCormick's cost estimates for apparatus were much too low, and that since much of the equipment needed for the laboratory must be made to specifications there would be long delays before operations could begin.[60] Since both Hammond and he were aware that the New York City purveyor's office was embarrassed by the long-standing debts owed to manufacturers,[61] Satterlee seemed to take particular satisfaction in cautioning Hammond that the laboratory would have to buy crude drugs on the market. If this were done with certificates of indebtedness, which sold at a discount to the disadvantage of the government, it would underline his contention that the government did not have sufficient funds to

pay cash for drugs, to say nothing of additional expenses involved in setting up new laboratories.[62]

Satterlee's objections to the laboratory might be attributed to
his conservative regard for traditional purveying policies, to his
own disappointment over his failure to secure the highest office
in the medical department, to his personal jealousy of Hammond,
and his distrust of Hammond's innovations. But beyond all these
motivations was another and perhaps more basic reason for what
seemed obstructionism—namely his close friendship with Squibb.

In 1858, Satterlee had induced Squibb to establish a pharmaceutical manufacturing laboratory in Brooklyn,[63] and from that
time on the army contracts received from Satterlee made up one
nucleus of Squibb's business.[64] To express his confidence in the
Squibb products, Satterlee wrote,

> . . . many of the chemicals and preparations which I supply
> habitually, namely those prepared by Dr. Squibb, cannot be
> had elsewhere except through uncertain channels and . . . I
> believe them to be better and more nearly officinal than
> similar preparations from other sources, and . . . uniform
> source of supply for the most important articles such as
> these, is desirable if not necessary to any good degree of
> uniformity in practice and results upon the sanitary condi-
> tion of the Army.[65]

Squibb's importance as a supplier of medicines to the army
sometimes was exaggerated, as when Frank Hastings Hamilton
noted in his treatise on military surgery that most of the medicines used in the United States army were produced in the
Squibb laboratory.[66] On the other hand, within three years after a
fire destroyed his laboratory (1858),[67] Squibb could repay bene-
factors who loaned him money to reestablish his business because, in Squibb's words, of the "preference given to a good
class of medicinal preparations by the Medical Department of the
Army."[68]

When the war orders came in, Squibb rented additional build-ings, and in 1862 purchased a site on which he constructed a new laboratory.[69] During the week ending April 18, 1863, there were forty-four employees on the Squibb payroll,[70] a force which was turning out all except a few preparations listed on the supply table in quantities equal to one-twelfth of all the medicines con-sumed by the army.[71] Most important were the panniers that were being filled as rapidly as the whole force of his establish-ment could produce them, not only for Satterlee but also (early in 1863) for the Philadelphia purveyor. One thousand of them were in preparation the last week in March 1863. By the end of that month, Squibb planned to complete delivery on orders for pan-niers totalling $40,000, and thereafter he hoped to receive further contracts for them to the value of $5,000 to $10,000 per week.[72]

Squibb, who was a member of the board that recommended improvements in the supply table during the summer of 1862, originated several articles found on the revised list of drugs—namely, a package of materials for preparing Ferri Oxidum Hydratum, a similar package for chlorinium, and a fluid extract of cinchona with aromatics, all of which he "placed entirely at the service" of the surgeon general's office.[73]

This cooperation notwithstanding, Squibb's relations with the government in 1863 were not as satisfactory as they had been earlier in the war. Various complaints from the army concerning his morphia induced him to conduct experiments in New York City hospitals to prove that his unbleached sulfate of morphia was the equal of bleached salts.[74] Such incidents[75] failed to shake the confidence of the surgeon general's office in Squibb's products. Indeed, there is no evidence that the Medical Depart-ment was dissatisfied with them because of qualitative consider-ations.

Yet by the autumn of 1862, Squibb remarked to the surgeon general that Jacob Dunton of Philadelphia had succeeded him "in a large share of the business . . . [he] at one time had of putting up

Army supplies."[76] This was especially true of a new type of pannier of Dunton, which differed somewhat from the Squibb pannier. The orders for panniers that Squibb was eager to fill in the spring of 1863 failed to materialize, for when Hammond inquired as to the price at which he could buy panniers of Squibb's pattern in Philadelphia, "equal in all respects to those now furnished by him," he was informed that T. Morris Perot & Co. and Hance, Griffith Co. would fill the panniers on more favorable terms than Squibb. Hammond's decision became still more unsatisfactory to Squibb, when an order went out to the Philadelphia medical purveyor to buy no more complete panniers, but to purchase the containers and prepare the "outfit" at the laboratory in Philadelphia.[77] Satterlee's observation that the Astoria laboratory could not "undertake a work . . . [such as the panniers] for some time yet," was not entirely reassuring to Squibb, who must have believed[78] that the competition of government laboratories would diminish his business.[79]

Squibb was further disgruntled by Hammond's choice for director of the Astoria laboratory. This was Charles McCormick, one of the most controversial surgeons in the army. In January 1863, he had just returned from New Orleans, where he had won Major General Benjamin F. Butler's accolade for the hospitals he organized and for other services he performed as medical director of the Department of the Gulf. In the flamboyant McCormick, Butler found a kindred spirit, hailing him as "the most competent medical director in the matter of yellow fever . . . in the country."[80] With the exception of one tour of duty (1842-1844), all of McCormick's posts from 1836 to 1858 were in the Gulf Coast region. He was stationed in New Orleans during the great yellow fever epidemic of 1853. In 1858 he went to San Francisco as medical director, remaining there until he took the field with the Army of the Potomac in November 1861. He was the inspector of hospitals in that army (December 1861 to February 1862), and after other brief assignments in San Francisco and at Fort Monroe, he went to Louisiana, but after Butler lost his command he came to New York City (December 1862).[81]

Disregarding the immediate fame which Butler, and to a lesser extent McCormick, won because of the sanitary measures in New Orleans, Squibb contended that McCormick was "but little more than a great quack, and . . . an unreliable man."[82] Earlier the two doctors had engaged in a running feud resulting from McCormick's report that "intelligent physicians" in the Army of the Potomac had complained to him that Squibb's opium was inferior in strength, assaying only 5 percent morphia compared to 9 percent in the McKesson and Robbins product.[83] Such claims were disproved by an analysis in the surgeon general's own laboratory where it was found that Squibb's opium was superior rather than deficient in strength,[84] but McCormick's underlings continued to repeat the accusations, even to a member of Congress, and in May 1863, Squibb finally requested that Hammond terminate McCormick's attacks upon Squibb's opium preparations.[85]

The quarrel between Squibb and McCormick was but one additional reason for Squibb and Satterlee to oppose the new laboratory at Astoria. Hammond either did not fully understand their attitude, or else chose to ignore it by ordering Andrew K. Smith to visit the Squibb establishment in preparation for his administrative duties in the Philadelphia laboratory.[86] When Hammond himself came to Brooklyn for discussions, Squibb argued that "the establishment of Army Laboratories might at . . . [that] time prove otherwise than economical or advantageous to the Government." After Hammond brushed aside the warnings as inconsequential, Squibb decided to convince Hammond by facts and direct observation. To this end he made the extraordinary offer that a responsible observer should be selected by Hammond to spend enough time in the Squibb laboratory to study the costs and other details of pharmaceutical manufacturing as a basis for a more thorough understanding of the problems involved in setting up the government laboratories. Considering that his employee, John Michael Maisch, was going to become the chief chemist in the Philadelphia laboratory, Squibb perhaps had little to lose in trade secrets when he proposed that Hammond's observer should have "free access to all details and operations of my laboratory." Yet, Squibb was known among the pharmacists of his day as a liberal sharer of scientific discoveries and techniques in the articles he spread on the pages of the *American Journal of Pharmacy* and elsewhere. In summarizing his offer of inspection to Hammond, he said,

> In order to arrive at a good basis for your final decision, I would suggest that one or more sound men and judicious medical officers be ordered for a month or more, to inspect closely the entire operations of my laboratory including the purchases, sources of supply, prices and stock of supplies necessary to be kept on hand; — the processes of manufacture, putting up, and packing; and the necessary qualities and qualifications in the way of buildings and apparatus and their cost. That this may be done as effectively as possible, I will expose to inspection all my bills, accounts and transactions freely, and will endeavour to place the officers you may send in such a position as may prevent their duty from being disagreeable to them. To obtain the best practical result they should be in the laboratory every day during the working hours, and keep notes which may be summed up at the close of their observations, and embraced in a concise report.[87]

After Squibb indignantly rejected Hammond's tactless suggestion that McCormick should be the medical officer to visit the Squibb laboratory on the extended inspection tour, Joseph H. Bill was ordered to New York City for that specialized service.[88] He remained in the Squibb establishment for several months, and in a comprehensive report to Hammond gave a description of the Squibb laboratory.[89] This report reveals, it seems clear, the näiveté of the young medical officer who obviously was given facts by Squibb to prove, first, that the Squibb manufacturing laboratory was capable of a sufficient increase in production to provide the government with abundant high quality medicines without any necessity for Hammond's experiment in state socialism, and, second, that the projected government laboratories would be unduly expensive from the standpoint of machinery costs and other outlays.[90] Bill, however, seemed to sense no ulterior motive, as he vigorously applied himself to his studies at the Squibb laboratory. He wrote to Hammond, "I have already availed myself of all the opportunities afforded me for obtaining information on the manufacturing of chemicals and have devoted the remainder of my time to a special study of the literature of the subject."[91] This concentrated effort probably gave Bill much of the preparation he needed when he became administrator of one of Hammond's laboratories less than a month after he finished his "course" with Squibb.

The manner in which McCormick began to organize the Astoria laboratory soon made him vulnerable to criticism. His order for the manufacture of bottle molds, for a type quite different from "the kind authorized or desired by the Surgeon General," brought him a rebuke in the form of a directive to cancel the order, with a further caution that "the bills for the same will not be paid by the Medical Department."[92] McCormick's first order for equipment included a small platinum basin for fusing silver nitrate, and a spatula of the same metal; he also wanted a silver jug and a bowl for caustic potash. Altogether his first requisition amounted to about $3,000. Prominent among the items were an ether still, eight furnaces, a set of five copper steam pans, and "an assortment of wooden, tin & zinc percolators" ranging in capacity from 5 to 100 gallons. Considering the scope of operations contemplated, this list did not in itself reveal extravagance. He requested only twenty-eight mattresses and twenty-one retorts.[93] Satterlee, however, commented to Hammond on the proposal to purchase "silver vessels," saying, "if I am rightly informed they can be dispenced with."[94] On the same day that Satterlee made his implied criticism of McCormick's "extravagance," Bill was reporting from the Squibb laboratory that in Squibb's "department of applied chemistry and pharmacy," there were no "platinum, silver or gold vessels . . . and in every respect the strictest economy consistent with efficiency is noticeable."[95] Squibb himself had already written in a letter to a friend,

> Dr. McCormick is just starting his [laboratory] at a great expense and under such circumstances that I predict for it a disastrous and disgraceful failure. . . . It is . . . a great pity that the best interests of the Medical Corps of the Army should fall into any such keeping.[96]

Delays in getting the Astoria laboratory into operation was another source of criticism. In an optimistic report made at the end of February, McCormick announced his intention of providing the New York City purveyor with drugs by the second week in March. The preparations, he predicted, would include from the beginning sweet spirits of nitre, the "different ointments and plasters," and after another week or so, chloroform.[97] Since the John Hyer Jr. firm that formerly occupied the laboratory buildings had manufactured chloroform, McCormick's forecast was not entirely impractical,[98] but there followed, during March, excuses for unforeseen delays.[99] When McCormick was finally relieved on May 25, he had spent $9,129.57 for apparatus, $1,564.96 for wages, and, in addition, $5,090 of quartermaster funds for fixtures, and lesser sums for transportation and rent, a total of $17,601.51.[100] But not an ounce of drugs had been produced there.

McCormick's administration at the Astoria laboratory was finally terminated by an episode that was not directly related to any dissatisfaction with his performance at the laboratory, but concerned his professional ethics prior to his appointment as director. Someone sent to Hammond during May 1863 a printed brochure written by McCormick under the title "Dr. Charles McCormick's Processus Integri or How To Use the Yellow or Magic Waverly pills," promoting a nostrum that McCormick himself had concocted.[101] Almost incredulous, Hammond sent an inquiry to McCormick, fully expecting the latter to declare that someone had been making unauthorized use of his name. McCormick, however, replied that he had written the memorandum printed for circulation with the pills. He admitted that he had caused the edition which Hammond had received to be printed when he had been stationed in San Francisco, but in his opinion he had violated no rules of ethics.[102] This brought a severe excoriation from Hammond,[103] and three days later Satterlee ordered Bill to relieve McCormick at the Astoria laboratory.[104] A medical board appointed to examine McCormick's conduct began its investigations in New York City,[105] and after weeks of waiting McCormick received orders to report to his "exile" in the Medical Department of West Virginia.[106] He refused to accept this assignment, but in 1864, when Hammond had been ousted and General Butler again held a field command, he once more appeared in Virginia as Butler's medical director in the Army of the James.

From correspondence between McCormick and Hammond it was evident that over a year before McCormick's removal "several members of the Corps" informed Hammond that McCormick had prepared "a secret medicine," which was sold by McCormick or his agents "under a quackish name"; but, according to Hammond, it was the advertising circular that precipitated the incident.[107] If Hammond did not receive his information from Squibb[108] or Satterlee, McCormick's departure from the Astoria laboratory was not regretted by either of them.

The future of the Astoria laboratory itself remained in doubt at the end of May. Andrew K. Smith approached Squibb with a proposal from the surgeon general to lease the Squibb laboratory to the federal government for one year. Under this rental agreement Squibb would have directed his laboratory with a commission as a surgeon of volunteers. Squibb, however, gave a negative reply:

> I have decided . . . that I cannot give up my permanent business for a temporary employment with the Government. Then, as I could not accept the management of the Laboratory for the Government, I could not rent it to be managed by others without building another in which to carry on my business, and the expiration of the Government lease would then make the large one [building] which now embarrasses me, still more of an embarrassment . . .[109]

Squibb then made a counterproposal, which included the following points:

1. To lease to the government "the ground or the real estate part of the property in question for the sum of one thousand dollars per annum, the Government to pay all the taxes and current expenses thereon." He included an option for the government to purchase the lot at the termination of the lease for ten thousand dollars.
2. Squibb "would sell the buildings, apparatus, fixtures, etc. except the books and a few personal articles, for the sum of ninety-five thousand dollars."
3. He also "would sell the manufactured articles on hand at ten per cent below the prices at which they have hitherto been supplied to the Army, and the unmanufactured material at the quotation prices of the wholesale market at the time of sale." The last items named he thought would amount to forty thousand dollars.
4. He would agree "to give half my available time during the first three months after the sale to superintending the Laboratory for the Government in conjunction with the officer who might be placed in charge of it, for the sum of one

hundred and fifty dollars per month, if it should be desired."[110]

Smith felt that since Squibb told him the establishment had cost between $55,000 and $60,000 the offer to sell for "$95,000 exclusive of ground rent," probably could not be entertained as a reasonable proposition.[111] At any rate, such an outlay would have required a special appropriation by Congress, which both Smith and Hammond well knew would be impossible with Stanton's influence arrayed against it. Smith, therefore, did not take the Squibb offer seriously, and Hammond agreed with him.[112] Uneasy though Squibb might have been over the future of his own business, it was evident that he would not part with it at a sacrifice.

Chapter 3

Obstacles and Achievements at the Astoria Laboratory

When McCormick made his controversial exit from Astoria, Hammond made a sound decision to appoint Joseph Howland Bill as medical officer in charge of the laboratory.[1] Although he was young (twenty-six on February 9, 1863), and never a pharmacist by profession, Bill had the advantage of a broad scientific education for those times. A Philadelphian by birth and upbringing, he received a baccalaureate degree at Princeton in 1855, and served for a season as an aide to Henry Wurtz, the state chemist and mineralogist, during a mineralogical survey of New Jersey.[2] When he began to prepare for a career in medicine, Bill studied in the office of his distinguished uncle, John Kearsley Mitchell, professor of surgery in the Jefferson Medical College, while he attended lectures at Jefferson. For clinical experience, Bill worked with his cousin, Silas Weir Mitchell, in the wards of a Philadelphia hospital. Professor Mitchell characterized his nephew as "an industrious student, of irreproachable character . . . unusually accomplished in chemistry, physics, mineralogy, geology, etc."[3]

In April 1858, Bill appeared before an army medical examining board. After passing that test, he began his career in the army as a contract surgeon and received his assistant surgeon's commission in 1860. The first year of the war found him in New Mexico where (in February 1862) he participated as a field surgeon in the engagement at Valverde in such an outstanding manner that his com-

manding officer cited his services by noting: "Assistant Surgeon
Bill in charge of the ambulances in the field was distinguished for
his energy and admirable arrangements for the relief of the dying
and care of the wounded." During the summer of 1862 he returned
to the states to administer an emergency hospital in Washington,
D.C., and then was sent to the second battle of Bull Run for
medical duty. Afterward, in Bill's words, he "returned at the heels
of the army" and followed it to South Mountain during the Antietam campaign. There he received orders to establish a hospital
(Hospital No. 3) at Frederick, Maryland, which he supervised until
he was directed (January, 1863) to take charge of another general
hospital in Cumberland, Maryland. These orders were cancelled
on February 11, because Hammond selected him for duty in New
York City.[4]

For a number of weeks following Bill's appointment to the
post formerly held by McCormick at Astoria, it seemed possible
that the laboratory would be discontinued before it could begin
operations.

To continue a policy of coordinating the two laboratories at
Philadelphia and Astoria, Andrew K. Smith exercised supervisory authority. He not only negotiated for the lease of the Squibb
establishment, but even before attempts to secure such an agreement failed, he recommended to Hammond that the Astoria laboratory should be abandoned, with Bill becoming assistant director of the Philadelphia laboratory.[5] As Smith listed them, the
disadvantages of manufacturing pharmaceuticals at Astoria were
numerous. It was inaccessible, nearly "six miles from the City
Park." It would be inconvenient to reach it from New York City
in the summer, and in the winter, with cakes of ice obstructing
navigation among the East River islands and at the Hell Gate, it
would become practically inaccessible to water transportation.
Its distance from the city would also make it difficult for employees to commute to work there, and the nearby suburbs could
not supply a sufficient working force. There was no running

water at the laboratory; wells had to be relied upon and the water forced into a tank. There was inadequate storage space and too few packing rooms or "accommodations for the female hands."[6]

In refusing to accede to Smith's suggestion that the government should give up the Astoria laboratory, Bill argued that most of Smith's criticisms were invalid. There was "a large brick warehouse" situated close to the laboratory building, and there were two frame buildings used for bottling. A supply of labor was always on hand which exceeded the laboratory's demand for it. The transportation of the finished preparations to New York City was troublesome, especially by way of the East River, but wagons also were available, although they were often drawn by "unserviceable horses" furnished by the Quartermaster Department.[7]

Hammond supported Bill, at least to the extent that he rejected Smith's suggestion that the Astoria establishment should be discontinued. On June 12, Hammond ordered that Bill should begin limited production—the "bottling of liquors and the preparation of powders, extracts, and tinctures," but other apparatus not required for those purposes was to be turned over to Andrew K. Smith if he requisitioned them.[8] The items authorized for production were similar to those on a list that Satterlee named the previous March when Hammond forced him to indicate what preparations he considered most feasible (or least objectionable) to make there.[9]

The bottling of wine, purchased in bond for army use, was soon under way,[10] but Bill still faced many obstacles. Smith continued as overall director of the laboratories, and—with Hammond deferring to his judgment on what articles should be produced at Astoria[11]—he recommended that operations be restricted to preparations requiring no further funds for apparatus.[12] This implied a concession to Bill's proposal that simple and resin cerates should be made,[13] as well as powders, extracts, aromatic spirits of ammonia, aromatic sulfuric acid, and citrine ointment. All other preparations were to be reserved for the Philadelphia laboratory.[14] A restricted program was required by the sheer fact that a portion of $200,000 allotted to the medical purveyors in Philadelphia and New York City to pay for "apparatus, raw material and expenses" of the laboratories, at Satterlee's suggestion, was diverted from the Astoria laboratory in June to settle other accounts. This included payments to contractors who had furnished supplies to the mishandled Banks military expedition of the previous winter.[15]

Even Bill's plea for "a small sum" to purchase testing apparatus brought no response from Washington for a time, although he offered to use his own analytical balance, which he had stored in Philadelphia. Without these essential instruments he could not perform assays on the incoming crude drugs or test the finished preparations.[16] Yet after a month, Satterlee, on orders from the surgeon general's office, sent brandy purchased from the Cozzens firm to Astoria for testing.[17] Bill then announced that he had "no apparatus sufficient for *any* analysis, chemical or pharmaceutical." He added, "I do not think it expedient . . . to make any large purchases of drugs until the analytical department is fitted up or to issue from the laboratory with its official label any medicines which have not been critically examined—without specific order to do so."[18] Late in August, only a few days before he left Washington, D.C., on an inspection tour to Hilton Head and the West, which was going to mark his separation from the surgeon general's office,[19] Hammond finally gave Bill permission to fit up the analytical department of his laboratory. But the cost of equipment was to be limited to about $500.[20] This consent was accompanied by an order to proceed with the production of cerates and preparations of iron.[21]

The limitations that Bill worked under still were not ended. That same month, Andrew K. Smith, acting upon the authorization given him in June to confer with Bill "in reference to the division of the Laboratory apparatus" at Astoria,[22] visited Bill's laboratory. The result was a decision to transfer two sets of chasers (burrstones) for milling operations to Philadelphia, together with apparatus for the preparation of Hydrargyrum cum Creta. The equipment was soon en route to Smith's laboratory.[23] Another incident suggestive of the circumstances was Bill's need to borrow from the Philadelphia laboratory 100 gross of one-quart bottles so that he might put up the wine and spirits that Satterlee had sent to Astoria.[24]

Other obstacles appeared when Bill found it virtually impossible, during the summer of 1863, to supervise in person the laboratory's operation except for a minor part of each working day. When he was given charge of the laboratory he was serving on the medical examining board in New York City, but he was not relieved of those duties and found that when the board was in session, he could not leave for Astoria in time to arrive there (in part owing to inconvenient steamboat schedules) until after 7:00 p.m.[25] A hospital steward, Frank Marquand, therefore was in "immediate charge," with the foremen, forewomen, chemists, and other civilian employees reporting to him each day. A second hospital steward carried out all the duties of inspection. The surgeon general's office even attempted to transfer Marquand, and only after considerable pleading was Bill able to retain his services during the early months of the laboratory's operations.[26] The other steward, however, was arrested after Bill detected him stealing opium.[27]

It was not until the middle of September that Bill was able to report that "All my arrangements are now complete . . . this Laboratory is at length prepared to manufacture all the articles of the supply table—with a few exceptions."[28] As he later admitted, Bill was still too optimistic; for although the work was "fairly commenced" the laboratory did not finally arrive at the degree of completion he claimed for it until February 1864. By that time he had spent for machinery, laboratory apparatus, and other equipment the sum of $11,744.10, in addition to the $17,601.51 expended by McCormick, and there were still orders outstanding that amounted to $2,200 for apparatus not yet delivered.[29] The cost exceeded Bill's earlier estimates, and doubtless also those of the Medical Department.[30] There was, nonetheless, an appearance of "the most rigid economy," an almost Spartan forbearance in expenditures. At the Astoria laboratory, Bill employed only a minimum of apparatus in his analytical department.[31] The Philadelphia laboratory printed its own labels from the beginning, but Bill's request for a printing press (cost $400) to do the same at Astoria was not granted until April 1864.[32] When the laboratory was producing at full capacity in the summer of 1864, Surgeon General Barnes rejected Bill's suggestion that a second medical officer be sent to him as an assistant.[33]

Bill collected a working force that varied between 100 and 200 persons. In February 1864, it was made up of one hospital steward, Frank Marquand, as general foreman; one hospital steward as inspector; two clerks (bookkeeper and shipping clerk); one errand boy; one superintendent of packing and bottling; one superintendent of packing and bottling liquors; two watchmen; five assistant chemists; thirty-six packers and bottlers; four forewomen; ninety women laborers; fifty-one boys and men laborers; and one engineer.[34] Except for the two hospital stewards, all those who were employed to work in the laboratory were civilians. The five men who were given the title "Assistant Chemist" prepared the medicines and won Bill's praise as "reliable and honest pharmaceutists." Three of them percolated the extracts, and one ground the powders and another was "exclusively occupied in compounding the pill masses." A crew of boys and adult laborers assisted them in the manual operations. Although he hoped to acquire one of the recently introduced pill-rolling machines that would turn out 500 pills each minute,[35] Bill had to rely upon fourteen of his women employees to convert the mass into pills with hand rollers.[36]

Because the bottling of liquors was a large part of the activity at Astoria, Bill assigned an especially reliable woman to test a sample, with an alcoholometer, from every barrel of incoming whiskey. He also directed that all wine received should be filtered to remove "an incredible amount of dirt and impurity." The processing of the liquors and alcohol was done in a separate building, by a crew of women under the supervision of a super-intendent and a forewoman, and so successfully that Bill observed with satisfaction, "Not a single case of drunkenness has occurred since I have had charge and the whiskey invariably runs over the guagers [sic] receipts."[37]

There was full employment, from 7:30 a.m. until 5:30 p.m., and from 7:00 a.m. to 6:00 p.m. during the summer months. In the autumn of 1863, the working day was for a time extended to midnight, with the additional hours credited to each employee as "an extra day's work." The average amount earned by each employee was slightly more than $1 per day, but Bill preferred a "piece work" system to a daily wage.[38] In the seven-month period ending in February 1864, the total man-days worked was 18,537; in that time $20,375.68 was paid out in wages.[39] After an increase in December 1863, the salary of the assistant chemists ranged from $50 to $75 per month.[40] Marquand's highest monthly stipend was $125.[41]

In administering the laboratory, Bill devised a system of receipts and invoices which, together with his elaborate devices for inspection, made an involved procedure. Whether or not this eliminated "fraud or habitual carelessness," at least it was designed to bring all the operations under Bill's scrutiny. As Bill described it, a specimen operation proceeded as follows:

A lot of opium comes to the Depot. The store keeper notifies the inspector of the fact and together they proceed to inspect and weigh it. If bad it is at once returned with the proper report. If apparently good it is weighed. The inspector gives the store-keeper a certificate that he has weighed and inspected this lot of opium noting the weight found. The inspector selects a sample from each case and then secures the opium in the cases in a safe place. He assays each sample of the opium and rejects all not containing seven per cent of Morphia. He now adds to the certificate given to the store-keeper a statement of the quality of the opium. If the opinion expressed is favorable, I order the storekeeper to receive the opium and it is transferred to his care. He files the inspector's certificate and enters the amount of the opium in a book (having a Credit and Dr. side) under the heading of "Gum Opium" and on the Dr. side of the book. When necessary he turns over the needed quantity of opium by weight to the miller (entering the quantity in the Credit side of his book) who receipts for the same. This person dries, powders, and bolts the quantity issued to him, and when this is done he notifies the inspector & hands him an invoice of the amount of powder obtained. If the operation has been properly conducted the inspector certifies the fact on the invoice and the powdered opium and the invoice are turned over to the store keeper. The invoice is filed and the amount of the powdered opium received entered into the book under the heading "Pulv. Opii" with the amount. The store-keeper at the same time issues the necessary bottles, corks, etc. to the chief filler who files the receipt. The bottles are then wrapped in hay, covered with paper, tied with twine, labelled on the outside of the package, and packed in boxes, each packer performing all these operations and recording his name in lead pencil on the inside of the box packed by him. On the outside of the box the name of the medicine, the date of the packing, and the source are stencilled. After nailing and strapping the boxes are turned over to the store keeper who enters their number and contents in a shipping book and at once despatches them to their destination, notifying the clerk, however, that the proper invoices may accompany them. The whole arrangement is so perfect that if at any time a purveying officer should complain that his opium is poor or badly packed he has only to examine the box, ascertain the date and the name inside, and *be definite* in his complaint to enable me to trace any error, fraud, or carelessness to the origin whether it arise from bad powdering, or careless filling or wrapping . . .[42]

The hospital steward who performed the duties of inspector was at least a ubiquitous figure in the laboratory. Beginning with his inspection of the crude drugs (he was supposed to conduct "three simultaneous assays" of opium, scammony, quinine, etc.), he was also ordered to keep a constant watch over "the several operations by which the crude material is converted into medicines," then to follow the medicines into the bottling room, and finally from there to the wrapping and packing division. After the preparation was ready to be issued, it was his duty to select four boxes for sampling, order them opened to examine the wrapping, quantities, and appearance of each bottle, and "in many instances" make assays of the contents. At no time, however, was this inspector to interfere in any way with the production. Only by rejecting raw drugs, by holding up the final order to issue them, or by reporting any "impropriety" to Bill could he exercise a positive check upon the processes.[43]

By the end of 1863 no less than eighty-three items listed on the supply table were being prepared for issue at the Astoria laboratory. Many of them were merely assayed and packaged, but others were processed or manufactured. Even the relatively simple processes—such as bottling and powdering—had often provided occasion, on an uncontrolled market, for drug adulterations. Some of the others, for example, the mixing of cerates, were deceptively simple, actually requiring as much care in trituration and other operations as the "nicer" preparations.[44]

The quantities of drugs ground and powdered with the granite milling apparatus (Bill's three sets of chasers and bedstones left to him after Smith's "raid"), a cast iron grinding mill for coarse powdering, and sieves of various meshes, were sufficient to push the apparatus to its capacity and keep the crews working overtime. Through December 1863, Bill's reports indicated that this equipment had turned out 162 pounds of ground blister beetles, 207 of ginger, 400 of licorice, 447 of cinnamon, 464 of cayenne, 469 of rhubarb, 504 of cinchona, and 651 of aloes. These, however, were all relatively small quantities compared to the 1,188 pounds of powdered squills, 2,200 of ipecac and opium (plus 789 pounds of ipecac and 1,204 pounds of opium ground separately), 2,940 of acacia, and 8,647 of black mustard.[45]

During the same first seven months of operation, the chemists made fifteen different fluid extracts in the percolators. Some of these, notably fluid extract of colchicum seed, were produced in nominal quantities and were experimental operations, but other extracts such as those of aconite root (611 pounds), valerian (817 pounds), senega (928 pounds), ipecac (1,063 pounds), and Prunus Virginianae (1,311 pounds) were made in quantity. In addition, fourteen tons of common cerate and 25,160 pounds of syrup of squills kept the open kettles filled many hours each day. There was also 6,632 pounds of laudanum and 500 pounds of tincture of ferric chloride, a small amount (213 ounces) of citrate of iron and quinine, 2,297 pounds of potassium iodide, 1,120 pounds of sodium bicarbonate, 2,693 pounds of cream of tartar, 508 pounds of potassium bicarbonate, and 8,870 pounds of compound spirit of lavender. It was evident that the earlier attempts to restrict the laboratory to a few of the simpler powders, extracts, and tinctures had been abandoned.

Imported crude drugs prepared for issue included asafetida, creosote, sulfur (1,015 pounds), copaiba (4,138 pounds), and camphor (6,424 pounds).[46] The acids which were transferred from carboys to bottles (but not manufactured at the laboratory) were aromatic sulfuric acid (1,744 pounds), dilute phosphoric, citric, tannic, and tartaric. Oils were also bottled, namely, cod liver oil (but only 960 quart bottles in the early months of operations), olive oil, oil of cinnamon, castor oil, and croton oil. In a separate building, a bottling crew dipped up spirits and wine from large wooden tubs into which they had been dumped from barrels and casks to fill 86,320 quart bottles of whiskey, 2,003 of brandy, 28,327 of sherry, and 31,020 of red wines (including port wine in this description).[47]

In 1864, twenty-two additional items were added to the list of the laboratory's products. Chloroform, which McCormick had promised in the spring of 1863, finally made its appearance. So did the solution of zinc chloride, Labbaraque's disinfecting fluid (chlorinated soda also used in the manufacture of chloroform), subcarbonate of bismuth, ammonia muriate, and liquid ammonia. Iodine also appeared on the list, but probably was packaged only, not prepared, as were alum, saltpeter, potassium chlorate, and lead acetate. There were also two additional extracts, those of cinchona and henbane. Muriatic, nitric, sulfuric, and acetic acids joined the acids already being prepared. Mercury ointment also was added to the list and, finally, four varieties of pills (compound cathartic pills, opium pills, pills of quinine, and camphor pills) were rolled in the laboratory. On the other hand, sixteen preparations which were put up or manufactured at Astoria before January 1, 1864, were not produced there after June 1, 1864, and fifty-two articles issued as materia medica through the major purveying depots during the war never were attempted at Astoria. On this list were such important preparations as ether, fused silver, Hoffmann's anodyne, liquid collodion, podophyllin, spirit of nitric ether, and essence of peppermint. All but eight of them were produced at the Philadelphia laboratory, indicating not only a policy of avoiding unnecessary duplication in the two laboratories, but also the greater diversity and extent of the activities at Philadelphia, and a greater confidence of the Medical Department's administrators, especially Surgeon General Joseph K. Barnes, in the Philadelphia establishment.

Production at Astoria was abruptly terminated, except for bottling and packaging operations, when fire swept through the laboratory on Monday morning, February 13, 1865.[48] After warnings from Washington that incendiaries might attempt to destroy the laboratories, and the consequent use of employees as watchmen to guard the buildings (at both Philadelphia and Astoria),[49] the Astoria fire was, ironically, accidental. Less than two months before the fire, Bill reported to Satterlee,

> The buildings are almost exclusively frame and fire is constantly apprehended, both accidental and intentional. To guard against the former five night watchmen are employed and a fire apparatus for extinguishing fire is at hand. Against the latter, a guard of five additional men selected by roster from among the male employees and armed with muskets are [sic] kept always on the alert being changed every twenty-four hours. Of course all this watching and guarding adds to the expense of the Dept.[50]

Notwithstanding these precautions, fire broke out in the ceiling of the drying room and spread rapidly throughout the laboratory, quickly reducing it to ashes. Bill's office was destroyed, and also some of the stock. One report of the damage set the government's loss at $50,000.[51] Operations continued in the other wooden structures at Astoria that were not consumed in the blaze, and the Philadelphia laboratory increased its output to meet the medical department's demand for drugs. Pharmaceutical manufacturers also were more than willing to take up the business. The *American Journal of Pharmacy* reported that in the two months following the fire, one firm received orders from the army to powder twenty-seven cases of opium, thirty-two ceroons of ipecac, eighteen ceroons of calisaya bark, 280 bags of cubebs, and other raw drugs in proportion.[52] Immediately after the fire, Barnes informed Satterlee that no steps should be taken to "reconstruct or re-fit the Laboratory," and that the "articles usually supplied by the Laboratory . . . [might] in the future be purchased without material delay or disadvantage."[53] Barnes could not forego the opportunity to let it be known that since, in his opinion, Hammond acted without adequate authority in establishing the laboratories, that he would decline to reestablish the Astoria facility without an act of Congress.[54]

Chapter 4

Operations at the
Philadelphia Laboratory

Without the friction that marked early developments at Astoria, operations began auspiciously at the United States Army Laboratory at Philadelphia (see Photo 4.1) late in April 1863, when Surgeon General Hammond ordered the Philadelphia medical purveyor to assign to it an allotment of Tarragona port for assay, bottling, and packing in wooden boxes.[1] Young women hired by the laboratory's director, Andrew K. Smith, processed this and the other large consignments of wine and spirits which followed it. Although it is notorious in the folklore of the Union armies that "medicinal whiskey" was at times diverted to other purposes, military medicine of the time prescribed huge quantities, much of it with quinine, but also for other uses in regular therapeutics. One shipment received at the laboratory in August 1863 consisted of 250 barrels of whiskey and 1,000 gallons of sherry.[2] Almost simultaneously with the first bottling operations the manufacture of pharmaceutical preparations began and accelerated rapidly after the first products were shipped, about May 1. Simple cerate, solution of ferrous tersulphate, ammonia liquor, blue mass, silver nitrate, and various powders were among the early items.[3] Moving ahead rapidly, Smith realized another of Hammond's objectives when he took with him to Washington, D.C., in July, four-ounce bottles of antimonial powder (James Powder), which bore the laboratory's new seal. These were the first experimental preparations of the laboratory.[4]

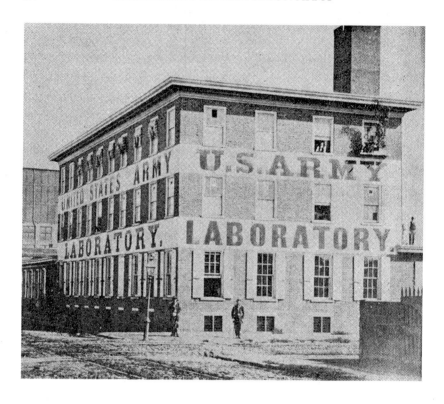

PHOTO 4.1. Main Building of the manufacturing laboratory at Philadelphia, where there was a larger operation than that established on Long Island, New York. Note the two military guards to the right of the gas streetlight. *American Journal of Pharmacy,* Vol. 75 (1903), p. 358.

On May 1, the monthly payroll was $341.81. But there was a steady increase after that, and by September 30 it had climbed to $3,736.11. The total amount spent for equipment, wages, and so forth to that date was $20,788.73.[5] Less than one-third of this was for "necessary apparatus and fixtures."[6] In addition to the steam engine and other machinery already in the building when it was rented, Smith's "scavenging operations" included the purchase from John Wyeth and Brother of "a great many things," including glassware, tin cans, jars, pots, and several thousand paper boxes that the Wyeths had stored in the building.[7] Smith procured scoops, sheet tin, enamelled kettles, cedar tubs, screw presses, chemical laboratory apparatus, sewing machines (for his hospital clothing department), and other articles from various suppliers.[8] Among the machines purchased there were two lathes for grinding glass stoppers, accompanied by "two artists" who operated them at the laboratory.

Most of the bottles were made from the laboratory's own mold in Pittsburgh, the "bottle headquarters" of America,[9] at nine dollars per gross for one-quart bottles (in 1863), a price much lower than that charged by glass manufacturers in Philadelphia.[10] The bottles, all with the impress "U.S.A. Hospital Dept.," were of various sizes, with a distinctive color and shape used to identify those which would contain poisons.[11] Labels bearing the laboratory's seal (see Photo 4.2) were pasted on all japanned-tin containers (see Photo 4.3) (similar to those of the Astoria laboratory) and packing boxes. Every bottle "of any size" not placed in a pannier or medicine wagon, was packed in a "square pasteboard box, surrounded with sawdust or rice husks." These were in turn securely fitted into wooden boxes for shipment.[12]

By September 30, 1863, $63,837.97 was spent on bottles, chemicals, and drugs.[13] Of this amount, $25,122.80 was for two large purchases from John Wyeth and Brother for articles that the Wyeths had previously stored in the laboratory building. On this list were 250 gallons of alcohol, 500 bottles of olive oil and castor oil, cerates, extracts, lint and bandages, knapsacks and panniers (of a type declared obsolete in 1863), and other materia medica "put up" at the laboratory during the early months of its operations. These were offered by the Wyeths to the government at a 10 percent discount from the usual wholesale price.[14] Some of the articles were found unfit for use by the laboratory; but after tests conducted by John M. Maisch indicated that the rest of them were of fair quality, they were issued.[15] The laboratory was

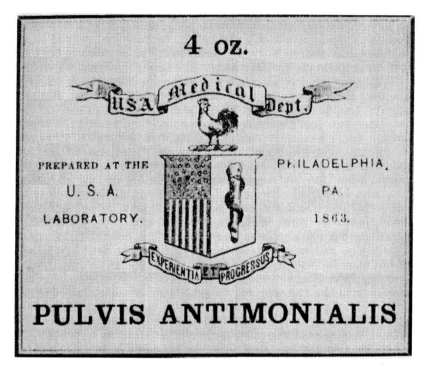

PHOTO 4.2. Label identifying a drug made at the laboratory in Philadelphia. It shows a shield with the stars and stripes and a sturdy staff of Asklepios. The ribbon motto beneath proclaims: "Experiment and Progress."

in this way brought into close relationship with John Wyeth and Brother, the pharmaceutical firm whose business with the Philadelphia medical purveyor already had been large, and whose dealings with the Medical Department later would become an issue in 1864. (Hammond faced court-martial on January 17, 1864, and was found guilty of exceeding his legal authority as Surgeon General and was forced to resign on August 22, 1864. An official inquiry in 1878 exonerated Hammond of all wrongdoing.)

In September 1863, after Hammond had begun the inspection tour from whence he would never return to the full duties of the

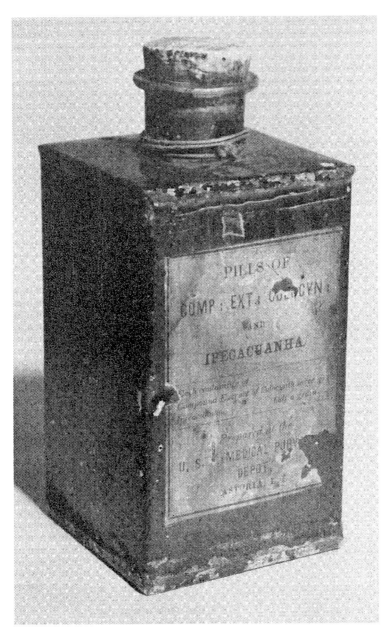

PHOTO 4.3. Crude metal container for pills, from medical purveying depot.

surgeon general's office, his successor, Joseph K. Barnes, noti-
fied Stanton that the Philadelphia laboratory was "in full and
perfect running order."[16] In general, the banishment of Hammond
meant that his enemies were going to be ascendent in the Medical Department.[17] Barnes, in particular, was always ready to
criticize Hammond's policies and did nothing to impede the
collection of unfavorable evidence against Hammond's administration of the Medical Department. Nevertheless, in a report to
Stanton after a rapid examination of Hammond's laboratories,
Barnes defended their objectives and praised "the present judi-
cious management of the Philadelphia laboratory." Barnes always tended to ignore the Astoria laboratory, but he noted that in
less than six months since it had begun production, the Philadelphia laboratory was already "producing a large proportion of the
chemicals and drugs required by the Army."[18] Again, in the
annual report of the surgeon general's office, Barnes wrote that
"even in its limited and experimental operations," the Philadelphia laboratory venture had proved to be "advantageous and
economical," and requested Stanton to seek "a small appropriation for additional machinery" needed.[19]

Whatever support Barnes gave to the Philadelphia laboratory
was more than likely due to the enthusiastic reports that Andrew
K. Smith sent to the surgeon general's office. When, in August,
the laboratory was just beginning to swing into full production,
Smith boasted, "we are daily increasing our facilities for
manufacture. . . . Our shipments are already more than one two-
horse wagon can haul, and I have recently been obliged to call
upon the Purveyor for transportation for his requisitions upon
me."[20] By the following December, he was able to list forty-
eight chemical and pharmaceutical preparations that were being
manufactured in the laboratory, in addition to extracts, tinctures,
powders, and pills. Beyond that, his filling department was "am-
ply large" to put up acids, gums, liquors, oils and hospital stores,
and such other articles as they did not manufacture. By then his

sewing department was manufacturing sheets, pillow cases, bed-sacks, pillow ticks, mosquito bar, towels, curtains, and was beginning to turn out hospital clothing. With trifling expense they might have produced chocolate and coffee extract![21]

A delay in the manufacture of Smith's ether and chloroform stills prevented the manufacture of chloroform until early 1864, but ether was being made at the laboratory before that. Tannic acid, sweet spirit of niter, and citrate of iron and quinine were other preparations not made until after 1863.[22] Smith was also mildly frustrated by a decision of the surgeon general's office to hold up his requisition for shafting, pulleys, and belting to put into operation the chasers and bedstones and other machinery that he had brought to Philadelphia from Astoria. Smith complained that for the lack of another bolting chest the sifting was often done by hand.[23] He was soon able to remedy these deficiencies in equipment,[24] however, and with the additional appropriation that Barnes got for him from Congress he continued to requisition new machinery in 1864.[25]

The rapid progress of the laboratory was due in no small measure to the aggressiveness of its director, the shrewd Connecticut Yankee Andrew Kingsbury Smith, a graduate of the Jefferson College of Medicine in 1849. He became an assistant surgeon in the United States Army, and from 1862 on was a major and surgeon.[26] Although his boasting, carelessness about submitting reports on time, and his occasionally ruthless conduct in dealing with his associates in the Medical Department denied him popularity among his colleagues,[27] he was an exceptionally able administrative officer.

Fully realizing that he did not possess the scientific knowledge essential to meet the technical demands of the laboratory, he was shrewd enough to obtain the appointment of John Michael Maisch as his chief chemist, and frankly admitted that it was from this brilliant master of pharmacy that he learned about the processes of drug manufacturing. To Maisch, in return, he gave a free hand in much of the planning, administrative supervision, and day-to-day control over the laboratory's operations.[28] So completely was this true that Martin I. Wilbert and others later had the incorrect opinion that Maisch was superintendent or director of the laboratory.[29] At least Smith's enthusiasm for Maisch was unbounded, as he wrote, "Mr. Maisch is a perfect jewel. . . . We did a big thing in getting Maisch—he is quiet, unassuming and industrious, and a perfect master of his business."[30] Maisch, in turn, expressed his confidence in Smith by declaring that "to the clear judgment and the uniform courtesy of this efficient officer" he mainly attributed his own success "in organizing the large establishment."[31]

Smith had not overestimated Maisch's abilities. The tall, genial young German (he was only thirty-two when he became chief chemist at the laboratory) had a "sunny, warm-hearted nature," but for all his kindliness he was a strong man, of "commanding appearance," with features that revealed his force of character. His "Teutonic thoroughness," sincerity, and inventiveness, his retentive memory, and his encyclopedic knowledge constantly impressed all who knew him or his work. "His brain," a contemporary wrote, "was a veritable chamber of facts and incidents relating to pharmacy and allied sciences, all systematically stored away or ready to quote at a moment's notice."[32] As Bullock pointed out, Maisch's was "a well-balanced mind."[33]

Maisch was prepared by education and training for his tasks at the laboratory. He was born at Hanau, the chemical manufacturing city on the Main, in Hesse, Germany, and there received training, especially at a new "Oberrealschule," in natural history, chemistry, mathematics, physics, and the "dead languages" (Latin, Greek). During his vacations he made botanical and mineralogical excursions through Germany. Because of his love for the microscope and original research in the fatty acids and resins under Bromeis at Hanau, he gave up his plans for the ministry and prepared for a scientific course at the university. When ill-

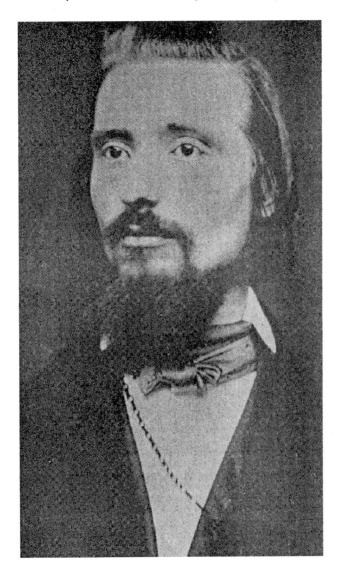

PHOTO 4.4. John M. Maisch at the age of twenty-six, a few years before he served the Union as the pharmacist in immediate supervision of the government's drug manufacturing laboratory at Philadelphia. At the end of the Civil War, Maisch became the first permanent secretary of the American Pharmaceutical Association. (As reproduced from an oil portrait. *American Journal of Pharmacy,* Vol. 75, 1903, p. 354.)

ness forced him to forgo a university education and, for a time, his prospective profession—pharmacy—Maisch came to the United States, after involvement with the Turners of Hanau in the Baden Revolution of 1849.

When he arrived in Baltimore, Maisch was almost penniless. He worked as a laborer in a box-making establishment and later in a mattress factory for a number of months. He then was able to find employment as a clerk in various pharmacies, first in Baltimore, then in Washington, D.C., Philadelphia, and New York City until the latter part of 1855, when for a time he worked in a chemical factory in Brooklyn.[34] In the meantime, during the 1850s, Maisch displayed chemicals of his own manufacture and won medals for them at exhibitions.[35] There also began, in 1854, the publication of his pharmaceutical articles in the *American Journal of Pharmacy,* the first of over 400 the journal would print before his death. A number of his early articles dealt with pharmaceutical manufacturing processes that were going to require skill at the United States Army Laboratory, for example, his careful packing of percolators in the manufacture of fluid extracts and a method for the preparation of mercurial ointment.[36]

In 1856, Maisch returned to Philadelphia to become employed as a pharmacist with E. B. Garrigues and Robert Shoemaker & Co., and, equally important for his later career, he soon was a most active member of the American Pharmaceutical Association. Several years later he was admitted to membership in the Philadelphia College of Pharmacy, to whose discussions and projects he made significant contributions.[37] Another professional opportunity became available in 1859 when the eminent Edward Parrish opened a preparatory school of pharmacy over his drugstore at 800 Arch Street, primarily for medical students who wished instruction in chemical science and pharmacy, and he invited Maisch to become an instructor. Parrish's colleagues in the American Pharmaceutical Association looked with some suspicion upon the new venture, even though Maisch, serving as a friendly intermediary, tried unsuccessfully to make the school a kind of annex to the Philadelphia College of Pharmacy.[38] Maisch announced his own courses, however, by newspaper advertisements. He also made for sale "Rare Chemicals not generally met with in commerce" in Parrish's laboratory and did chemical analyses to order.[39] While he was at Parrish's school and later, Maisch helped his employer to revise *Parrish's Introduction to Practical Pharmacy,* which is considered the first truly American textbook of pharmacy. One revision appeared in 1859, and a much more significant rewriting of it came out as Parrish's *Treatise on Pharmacy,* Third Edition, in 1864.[40]

In September 1861, after two years with Parrish, Maisch became Professor of Materia Medica and Pharmacy in the College of Pharmacy of the City of New York, where he remained until he received his appointment at the United States Laboratory in 1863.[41] Receiving a salary of only $300 per annum, and with lectures only three evenings each week,[42] Maisch was able to continue his own pharmaceutical investigations, to publish numerous articles,[43] and to accept part-time employment in the Edward R. Squibb manufacturing laboratory in Brooklyn.[44] This practical experience in Squibb's establishment, at a time when Squibb was producing large quantities of medicines for the United States Army, probably was the most valuable preparation that Maisch could possibly have received for his position in the government laboratory.

Maisch agreed to become chief chemist at the laboratory for a salary of $1,500 per year.[45] When Smith secured a wage increase for his employees, in April 1864, there was a $300 raise for Maisch.[46] That was the only change until rising living costs and the expenses of a family forced Maisch to request more compensation in December 1864. Smith and Murray then tried to win not only a salary adjustment but a measure of prestige for their chief chemist and "foreman," by securing for him an appointment as a surgeon in the United States Army. The surgeon general bluntly refused this,[47] even though, as Murray reminded him, a similar offer of a commission as surgeon of volunteers had been made "to an eminent chemist of New York City," meaning, of course, Squibb.[48] Following Barnes' action, Maisch threatened to resign his position, and again Smith strongly supported him. He wrote to Barnes, "His reason is simply this—He has received offers of employment at a much larger salary than his present pay, and upon this amount he is unable to live and support his family, without running into debt. This salary is now $1800 per annum. It is with him a question of dollars and cents."[49] After this explanation, Smith asked that Maisch's salary be increased to $3,000. Barnes then recommended $2,300 and Stanton approved it.[50]

When the Philadelphia laboratory was running at full capacity, it employed over 350 women in its filling and sewing departments alone.[51] These, together with chemists, artisans, common laborers, hospital stewards, and supervisory personnel, made a much larger working force than at Bill's establishment in New York City. Maisch's departments were administered by brilliant young civilian pharmacists who moved on to responsible positions in the pharmaceutical manufacturing industry after the war. The laboratory was, in fact, an important in-training experience for young men who were able to grasp the significance of pharmacy in connection with the new industrialism that the war was helping to bring into being.

One of the most brilliant protégés of Maisch at the laboratory was C. Lewis Diehl. Like Maisch, he was born in Germany (at Neustadt, in the Rhenish Palatinate, Bavaria). He graduated from the Philadelphia College of Pharmacy in 1862, enlisted in the Fifteenth Pennsylvania Volunteers, was wounded at Stone's River, and discharged from the service in 1863. He left the laboratory in 1865 and went to Louisville, where he reorganized the Louisville Chemical Works. For twenty-eight years he was a powerful influence in the development of the *National Formulary*.[52] Another of Maisch's young pharmacists, Henry W. Scheffer, in charge of the steam laboratory (i.e., the main operations room), was later a member of the St. Louis firm of Larkin & Scheffer.[53]

There were also young hospital stewards at the laboratory. One of them, Henry H. Jacobs, was Philadelphia-born, a graduate of the Philadelphia College of Pharmacy (1862), and just beginning his career as a pharmacist when he enlisted as a hospital steward on April 18, 1863, and was assigned to the laboratory on May 4, 1863.[54] He was the first with that rank to serve there, but he was followed on July 11, 1863, by William J. Scott;[55] Charles L. Cummings;[56] and William H. Webb, another Philadelphia pharmacist, who enlisted as a hospital steward on October 7, 1863, for five years and was transferred to the laboratory in 1864.[57] Chapman H. Evans, Victor Abadie, and Stephen F. Peckham of the Seventh Rhode Island Volunteers arrived early in 1865 to take charge of the important ether and chloroform department, a position previously filled by the son of Dr. Hartshorne, a prominent advisor to the surgeon general's office.[58] At the end of the war, Peckham was in turn relieved by Augustus Henkel, another young German druggist who enlisted as a hospital steward on September 28, 1864.[59] Not all the stewards were efficient, and when they failed to measure up to Maisch's exacting requirements their transfer was requested. One such person was characterized (the words were almost certainly those of Maisch) as "a lazy, worthless fellow, a careless breaker of apparatus and a mere dabbler in chemistry."[60] In general, however, they were men of ability and when the civilian chemists left the laboratory late in the war (as did Hartshorne), their places were taken by the hospital stewards.[61]

There were also important administrative changes that affected the laboratory late in the war. Robert Murray, as medical purveyor, always supported Maisch, and allowed both Smith and

Maisch considerable autonomy in administration, while accepting responsibility for the laboratory's policies as an adjunct of his purveying depot. When his appointment as successor to George E. Cooper became one of the storm centers in the Hammond affair, it is reasonable to suppose that his position in Philadelphia became increasingly uncomfortable. In December 1863, an order was drawn up transferring Murray to San Francisco, but this was cancelled.[62]

The laboratory was probably no more of a problem than his other duties, but nonetheless Murray's relations with Smith were increasingly troublesome. He had the last word on hirings and dismissals at the laboratory, but the personnel were actually being selected by Smith and Maisch.[63] His accounts also became increasingly involved because he was instructed to open an entirely separate account on his books for the laboratory. It was charged with the raw materials it consumed, labor costs, and other expenses, and credited with "all supplies furnished . . . ready for issue." This meant that crude drugs and other articles used by the laboratory were procured by the medical purveyor and issued (with written forms) to the director of the laboratory. When the manufactured articles were turned over to the purveying depot they had to be formally issued by the director to the purveyor. The articles appeared on the records of the purveyor's office twice; once before they were prepared and again when they were ready for shipment, with invoices and receipts constantly passing back and forth.[64] It was not until January 1865, that the director of the laboratory was finally authorized to receive crude drugs and other supplies that were delivered by the suppliers directly to his establishment, and to sign receipts for them. By then even Satterlee was using a similar procedure in New York City.[65]

Several incidents led to personal friction between Murray and Andrew K. Smith. One of these occurred over what Murray considered a strategem of Smith's to use testing of spirits at the laboratory as a device to give the liquor business of the purveying depot to merchants favored by the laboratory director.[66] This matter became more serious when Murray incorporated it in his testimony against Hammond at the Hammond trial in 1864. There were other clashes, for example, when Murray characterized as "groundless" charges of disloyalty made by Smith against the forewoman of the laboratory's sewing department.[67] As a culmination of these disputes, changes were made in the administration of the purveying depot and the laboratory.

In October 1864, the duties of the Philadelphia medical purveyor's office were divided between Murray and F. A. Keffer.[68] The latter was made responsible for the public property at the depot (including, presumably, the laboratory property) and Murray retained control of the public funds.[69] Soon thereafter, Andrew K. Smith received orders that relieved him from duty at the laboratory and reassigned him to Major General William T. Sherman's command as medical director of the Department of South Carolina.[70] There was some delay in this transfer, however, because Murray did not wish Smith to leave until his accounts and other affairs were "properly arranged."[71] In January 1865, with the explanation that Smith's services with Sherman's army were "not required," the special orders that had directed his transfer were revoked, and Smith was allowed to remain as director of the laboratory.[72] Before that decision was reached, however, the obvious move to make Keffer director of the laboratory had been considered.[73] Meanwhile, Murray was relieved of his duties as medical purveyor and sent to San Francisco.[74] He was replaced by Charles McDougall, medical director of the Department of the East.[75]

Administrative changes influenced the Philadelphia laboratory very little as it continued to turn out medicines for the armies. In contrast to Bill's "miserable collection of sheds" at Astoria, its facilities for manufacturing drugs and chemicals compared very favorably with the other pharmaceutical laboratories of that day.

If anyone, for example, should have come to the government
laboratory after an inspection of the Charles Ellis Son & Co.
establishment in the same city, he or she would have seen much
the same kind of apparatus—steam-operated grinders and stirring machines, filter presses, sand and water baths, jacketed copper pans, percolators, stills, and even an elevated drying room
that compared to that of the Ellis firm.[76] Because Edward
R. Squibb generously published drawings of his inventions in the
pharmaceutical periodicals,[77] and because Maisch knew the Squibb
laboratory thoroughly, the equipment and technologic innovations at the Philadelphia laboratory closely resembled those of
Squibb. Procter noticed that this was true of the oscillating machine for mercurials (blue pills, mercurial ointment, etc.) and the
ether apparatus.[78] He might have added other similarities such as
the procedures followed in making chloroform, heavy oil of
wine, and in percolation. Diehl later wrote that all the methods of
manufacture and the apparatus employed were essentially the
same "as those then practiced and in use in the laboratory of
Dr. E. R. Squibb."[79] Early in the laboratory's development, however, Procter noticed that the plan of one device that Squibb had
inspired was "more simple" at the laboratory.[80] In this piece of
apparatus, in the "oleum aethereum" process, and in other ways,
Maisch and his staff by their own inventiveness improved upon
some of the Squibb machines and processes.

The main building of the laboratory group stood "flush with
the pavement" facing west on Sixth Street, and extended northward from the intersection of Sixth and Oxford Streets for about
100 feet. It was brick, three stories high, with a brick-floored
basement.[81] Upon entering from Sixth Street, a visitor to the
laboratory arrived in a narrow hallway. To the left, doors led to
the director's office, and next to it was Maisch's office, which
was fitted up as an experimental laboratory. It was there that
Maisch tested the crude drugs and chemicals, and carried on his
private research.[82]

To the south of the corridor was the storekeeper's room for receiving, storing, and making available when needed the glassware, tinned containers, panniers, packing boxes, and other equipment.[83] From this room, proceeding southward, one next came to the milling room, where the raw drugs were ground into coarse or fine powder and bolted. The apparatus in this room included the oscillating machine for mercuric pill masses and other preparations of free metallic mercury, a Bogardus mill, chasers and bedstones (some of these were acquired from Astoria), and bolting machines. From the milling room fine powders such as ipecac, jalap, rhubarb, and others were taken by an outside stairway to a second-story room for packaging. The drugs ground for percolation were sent directly to the steam operating room.[84]

Directly over the mill room, on the second floor of the main building, there was the filling room, where the dry materials—powders, salts, and pills—were bottled and packaged. Eventually 150 women, supervised by a forewoman, were employed in this department. Women using hand-operated pill machines rolled the various kinds of pills.[85]

During the laboratory's first months the north end of the second floor was used as a sewing room with twelve women turning out hospital linens and roller bandages. Operating about ten sewing machines, they made sheets, pillowcases and towels.[86] By the end of 1863, bed ticks, mosquito bar, and curtains were added to the list of products,[87] and the government authorized Murray to begin the manufacture of hospital clothing.[88] The sewing department was instituted as a part of Hammond's plan for the laboratory. From his personal experiences as superintendent of the Wheeling General Hospital early in the war, the surgeon general knew that the hospitals had been receiving insufficient quantities of these hospital supplies from the Medical Department—and sometimes none at all.[89] Within a short time after he began these operations, Smith found it necessary to expand his staff so rapidly that the room on the second floor of the main building was inadequate. He then moved the entire sewing department (eventually there were 250 women and girls employed in it) to the second floor of the other building, which he acquired for the laboratory at Sixth and Master Streets.[90]

The third floor of the main building was occupied by a filling room for fluid extracts and other liquid preparations (except spirits) that were bottled, labeled, and then temporarily stored on shelves above the work benches. Girls were employed at nearby sinks washing bottles,[91] but a wash house for bottles was also operated later in another building. There was also a scaling room on the third floor. One man was stationed there to paint a solution of citrate of iron and quinine on panes of glass. After allowing them to dry in a warm closet he would scrape off flakes of the drug with a spatula.[92] Another employee made isinglass plaster by mixing isinglass, benzoin, and water, and then applying the mixture with a brush to silk that was stretched on a frame. After several successive coats were applied to the black or flesh-colored cloth, the reverse side of the fabric was backed with a mixture of venice turpentine and tincture of benzoin.[93]

A number of women worked in the brick-floored basement of the main building, bottling liquors and wine.[94] After the laboratory's products were packed in the panniers, knapsacks, or wooden boxes for shipment, they were taken in drays to the Sixth and Master Street building, and there stored on the first floor of that warehouse until they were requisitioned by medical purveyors.[95] Some of the drugs, however, were put directly into new medicine wagons, especially those of the Autenrieth pattern.[96]

Adjoining the south end of the main building at a right angle, there was a one-story brick structure that ran eastward along Oxford Street. This was the steam laboratory room, or still room as Maisch called it. The interior length was 56' 3", and from north to south it was 39' wide. There was a brick floor and nine windows which, together with open transoms above the doors, provided the only ventilation. A short flight of stairs led up to the mill room. Built against the east wall of the main building and jutting into the northwest corner of the steam laboratory was a brick boiler room ($26' \times 10'\ 3''$).[97] Above the boiler room, and having the same dimensions with a $9'$ ceiling and skylight, there was a drying room where opium and other drugs were dried before being powdered in the mill room. An engine room, separated from the steam laboratory by a wooden partition, was located directly to the east of the boiler room. It contained a twenty-five horsepower steam engine that drove the grinders and other machinery. The steam boilers, in addition to providing the steam for the stillroom, also heated the drying room and the main building.[98]

Efficient planning governed the distribution of apparatus in the steam laboratory room. The large percolators, made of wood with tinned-copper linings, were placed upon a raised platform at the west end of the room on a level with the mill room from where they received granulated and pulverized drugs. Procter noticed that their capacity ranged from 150 to 260 gallons, and that they were packed with 280-pound charges of colocynth and 600 pounds of valerian in single operations.[99] After the displacement process was completed, the refuse was easily removed from them through clean-out holes located at the front and near the bottom of each percolator. Another detail that came to Procter's attention during his tour of the stillroom once more demonstrated how Maisch reduced the operations of the laboratory to a system. Procter reported, "Hanging in front of each percolator is a blackboard, on which is written the leading facts of each operation as they are developed, such as name and quantity of material, menstruum, and percolate, with remarks when necessary."[100] Fourteen different fluid extracts were prepared.

In addition to the percolators, the steam laboratory contained apparatus for distillation, evaporation, crystallization, washing, and decantation. From them came fluid and solid extracts, numerous salts, ammoniacal products, and others. A row of jacketed steam evaporators and stills stood at the east end of the room. The copper kettles were almost certainly the type used by Squibb, quickly heated by forcing steam between the inner and outer layers of their double bottoms and equipped with still-heads, which converted them into retorts. To recrystallize salts, wash precipitates, and for other purposes, large tanks were required (capacity up to eighty gallons). These, like Squibb's, must have had block-tin linings and double walls into which steam could be injected.[101]

Although steam was essential in the manufacture of chloro-form and ether, a tall shed located a short distance from the steam laboratory housed the stills used in preparing them.[102] Hammond authorized the erection of this "ether-house" in May 1863,[103] despite a warning from the quartermaster general that a new city ordinance forbade the construction of temporary wooden build-ings.[104] The chloroform still went into operation in 1864.[105] Sweet spirit of niter (342,642 ounces total) also was made there. As a precaution against fire, steam was piped in from the boiler room, and no flame was permitted within the building. Combus-tible products were bottled and stored in its underground store-room.[106]

The laboratory buildings were on a rectangular piece of ground, $150' \times 175'$. In the early months of operations a fence marked the eastern boundary of the lot line. But as the laboratory expanded, a frame building replaced the fence and extended across the property from north to south.[107] It was a series of rooms: a stoppering room where the bottle stoppers were shaped; the washhouse for cleaning the bottles sent into the laboratory; a tin shop; and a carpenter shop.[108] North of the main building there was another detached building. Like the steam laboratory, it was one story high and made of brick. Beginning at Sixth Street, it followed the northern boundary of the laboratory site eastward for nearly 100 feet. The eastern fifty feet of it contained the important furnace room,[109] where, as Maisch described it, "preparations were manufactured by the aid of fire."

The furnace room's central feature was a large free-standing chimney, surrounded on four sides by as many furnaces stoked with anthracite coal. One of them was hooded. In the southeast corner, another chimney stack had a flue that connected with a furnace outside the building. Wooden tanks lined the north wall, and others of solid lead for the sulfuric acid mixtures were in a row along the east wall. The work table stood against the west partition, and under the windows at the south side of the room there were sinks and shelves for glassware, crockery, and other small apparatus. Even in this room open windows and doorways provided the only protection from dangerous fumes except for the one hood and the flues. The ceilings were high, there was sufficient natural light, and the floor, as in the stillroom, was bricked. C. Lewis Diehl, the superintendent of the department, performed most of the operations with the help of one assistant, a young and intelligent laborer, with other laborers brought in for special tasks.[110]

Diehl employed open vessels in making a number of his preparations. There was, for example, a crane in the furnace room (see Photo 4.5) that swung large enamelled kettles over one of the fires, heating vinegar of squill, and sugar for Syrup of Squill. The solution was then strained while it was still hot.[111] Another large kettle was used to prepare solutions of sodium carbonate, potassium carbonate, and other saline compounds.[112] Quinine and a citrate of iron solution were heated in a water bath at 120°F until the quinine was dissolved. The solution was then evaporated to a consistency of a syrup, placed in earthenware jars, and taken to the scaling room on the third floor of the main building to be spread on plates of glass for drying.[113]

Citrine ointment, prescribed for chronic skin diseases, ulcers, and irritations of the eyelids, was produced in quantities of fifty pounds or more at a time by heating neatsfoot oil and lard in an

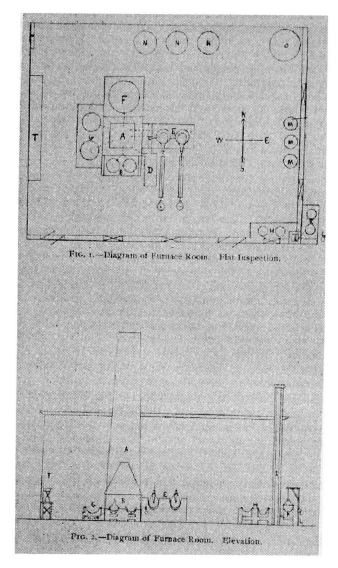

Fig. 1.—Diagram of Furnace Room. Flat Inspection.

Fig. 2.—Diagram of Furnace Room. Elevation.

PHOTO 4.5. Furnace room where pharmaceutical operations requiring heat were carried out at the Astoria laboratory. Key to diagrams: A—central stack; B—hooded furnace; C—vaporizing tube; D—condensing chamber; E, F, G—furnaces; I—stack; H, K—furnaces; L—crane; M—solid leaden tanks (for sulfuric acid mixtures); N—wooden tanks; T—work table; W—wardrobe. (*American Journal of Pharmacy*, Vol. 78, 1906, p. 562.)

earthen vessel to 200°F, removing it from the fire, and adding mercury dissolved in nitric acid.[114] Instead of stirring this with a spatula, the chemist employed an agitator developed by Squibb.[115] To make lead plaster, litharge in fine powder with olive oil and water were boiled in an open kettle. Diehl then rolled out the sodden mass upon a marble slab before macerating it in a trough of cold water, and allowing it to harden in the air.[116] The relatively primitive nature of these pharmaceutical operations is illustrated in the manner of preparing Monsel's solution. Diehl would take a large enamelled kettle to a small wooden shed outside the furnace room, and there would oxidize ferrous sulfate with nitric acid so that the fumes could escape without the use of a hood.[117]

Many of the most important operations employed covered capsules and other receptacles of porcelain, iron crucibles, and tubulated glass retorts heated on shallow sand baths. Potassium carbonate and potassium acetate were both evaporated to dryness in shallow dishes before one of the furnace openings. The latter preparation, while still hot in the furnace room, was filled into wide-mouthed bottles. Diehl also evaporated mercuric nitrate in a sand bath and triturated it until he obtained "beautiful bright-red crystals" of mercuric oxide.[118] Potassium permanganate, suddenly in demand as a disinfectant and for local application to hospital gangrene lesions, ulcers, and abscesses, was processed in the furnace at the southeast corner of the room. There the caustic potash, black oxide of manganese, and chlorate of potash with dilute sulfuric acid and distilled water were evaporated over a sand bath, then placed in a covered Hessian or Cornish crucible and heated for an hour, until a semifused mass was formed.[119]

Benzoic acid, mainly employed in camphorated tincture of opium, was produced by heating benzoin with a conical paper cap held over the receptacle until the rising vapor could be trapped in the cone.[120] After making mercuric sulfate by the direct action of sulfuric acid on mercury, Diehl mixed the sulfate with sodium chloride and transferred it one spoonful at a time into a tubulated retort (a "sublimation" or vaporizing tube), which was heated over a sand bath. Mercuric chloride then passed into a unique condensing chamber (see Photo 4.6) that consisted of a series of shelves open at alternate ends so that the vapor would pass back and forth, drawn by the draft of the flue, depositing corrosive sublimate as fine powder on the shelves as it did so. Sodium sulfate accumulated in the retort and was occasionally scraped off.[121]

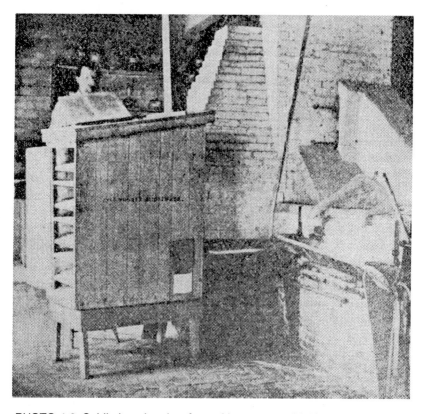

PHOTO 4.6. Subliming chamber for making mercury bichloride, as used in pharmaceutical laboratories during the Civil War. (*American Journal of Pharmacy,* Vol. 78, 1906, p. 567.)

Tincture of ferric chloride was a new officinal preparation during the Civil War, prescribed as a powerful hemostatic. Diehl manufactured it in two stages. First, he prepared ferrous chloride by the action of muriatic acid on card teeth, then heated the ferrous chloride with nitric acid. The solution of ferric chloride was mixed with alcohol in the filling room, at a ratio of 1 to 3, and put into stoppered bottles.[122]

After considerable breakage of funnels and loss of phosphorus, Diehl deviated from the official directions for the preparation of dilute phosphoric acid by returning to the older method of oxidizing the phosphorus. In a French glass tubulated retort, he would combine twelve parts of water and two parts of phosphorus, then "place the retort on a sand bath and introduce through a funnel tube, fixed in the tubular by means of a cork and reaching half an inch below the level of the liquid, eight parts of nitric acid. Heat was then applied to the retort, and when the reaction began to slacken he added more nitric acid."[123] One of the most exacting and difficult operations in the furnace room, and one in which Diehl and Maisch doubtless took the most pride, was the distilling of heavy oil of wine from alcohol and concentrated sulfuric acid in large retorts (6½ to 7 gallon capacity) set in a deep sand bath with the furnace flues carefully adjusted to keep the temperature within a narrow range and prevent frothing over. The heavy oil of wine collected in a receiver and was converted into Hoffmann's Anodyne.[124]

Not all of the processes in the furnace room required direct heat. In one of the steps required to make citrate of iron, iron hydroxide was precipitated into a large wooden tub. Likewise, chlorinated lime mixed with sodium carbonate in a tub which had a capacity of 300 gallons, gave chlorinated soda.[125] After immersing cotton in potassium nitrate and sulfuric acid, the mixture was carefully stirred, put in large stoneware jars, and allowed to stand for twenty-four hours to produce collodion.[126] And, working at his bench, Diehl converted silver nitrate, which he had made on a sand bath,[127] into small, fused, cone-shaped masses (Argenti Nitras Fusus) by melting it in a dish with the flame of a Bunsen burner and then pouring it into molds.[128]

John M. Maisch combined a pragmatic interest in the operational problems of the laboratory with his own scientific investigations. In 1863, a small library purchased with $200 of Medical Department funds, and a yearly allocation of $100 after that, permitted him to keep reference volumes in his laboratory.[129] More important than this, he continued to read German chemical and pharmaceutical periodicals. He even found time to submit significant translations of extracts from them to the *American Journal of Pharmacy* for republication,[130] and applied the findings of the Europeans to the specific processes of the laboratory. In the production of heavy oil of wine, for example, Maisch compared his own results with those of Kuhlman, Marchand, Lose, Mitscherlich, and Duflos. Diehl helped him by keeping accurate statistics, and made suggestions for a method of reheating the retorts, which kept temperatures between 302°F and 315°F. By careful manipulation they were able to increase the yield of oil to 5.52 ounces from 157 ounces of sulfuric acid and 71.77 ounces of alcohol, compared to Squibb's average of 4.54 ounces from 173 and 111 ounces respectively of sulfuric acid and alcohol.[131]

Maisch's inventive genius was also much in evidence. The successful bolting machine, which relieved the employees in the mill room of hand-sifting tasks, was an improved design of Maisch's invention.[132] On the third floor of the main building the movable frame, on which the isinglass plaster was stretched, was the simple but effective product of Maisch's ingenuity. It was manufactured especially for the laboratory by A. H. Wirz of Philadelphia.[133] Instead of preparing zinc sulfate in the usual manner, directly from zinc, Maisch developed a less expensive process in which zinc white was dissolved in sulfuric acid, then evaporated and crystallized.[134] Perhaps the most significant of his contributions, however, was his invention of the sublimation tube and condensing chamber for the manufacture of corrosive sublimate. This departed radically from the usual procedure of subliming the vapor into crystalline masses, although it was similar to the method used up to that time in the manufacture of sulfur and quicksilver.[135]

Maisch's interest in pharmaceutical botany also remained keen at the laboratory as he continued to work on a formula for fluid extract of colchicum. He was able to report that he produced experimentally at the laboratory six pints of the oil from 118 pounds of the seed. After tests of incoming *Veratrum viride,* which had dead stalks, roots, and corms attached to it, he concluded that the stalks contained no alkaloids and ordered his chemists to remove them before charging the percolators.[136]

Many of the basic drugs and chemicals of the laboratory were purchased through Harrison Smith, a Philadelphia drug broker with forty years experience, who was purchasing agent for John Wyeth and Brother at the time that it was supplying the Medical Department with a major part of the medical preparations it bought in Philadelphia.[137] Here was another of the numerous links between the laboratory and John Wyeth and Brother during the Hammond regime. In his dealings with the laboratory, however, Harrison Smith did not reveal a marked bias in favor either of John Wyeth and Brother, or any other firm. The first orders for raw drugs went to Dix & Morris, Schieffelin, and Rosengarten and Sons. By the end of May 1863, no less than sixteen drug firms shared the laboratory's business, with the largest orders going to Powers & Weightman, Schieffelin, and Charles Pfizer & Co. Among the purchases was one for $756 from Philadelphia bankers Jay Cooke and Company, for silver. By the end of September 1863, the medical purveyor's office had dealt with no less than twenty-nine firms on the laboratory's account.[138] Murray also purchased some of the drugs (without paying a commission on them to Harrison Smith) directly from samples submitted to the medical purveyor's office. On occasion he found himself obliged to beg other purveying depots for scarce drugs, such as opium, when the supply of the laboratory was nearly exhausted and the market price was exorbitant.[139]

Medical storekeepers and purveyors received instructions to forward to the Philadelphia laboratory any medical or hospital supplies accumulating at their depots that were not on the current supply table, and indeed a motley variety of drugs were sent in from the different warehouses. Among them were fluid extracts of columbo and dandelion, subnitrate of bismuth, chamomile flowers, gum opium, and (after Hammond's order dropping them from the table) calomel and tartar emetic.[140] It was, of course, the surgeon general's intention that the laboratory, so far as possible, should use them in the manufacture of officinal preparations. According to Murray, many of them were disposed of either in that way or in experimental operations. Whenever they could do it, Maisch and Smith (through the purveyor's department) bought indigenous drugs directly from firsthand suppliers, such as the plant collectors who came to the laboratory offering botanicals for sale. In discussing this practice, Smith wrote:

> Many of the vegetable productions made use of in the preparation of our medicines can be purchased by me from my countrymen at a far less rate than [that] charged by wholesale druggists. For instance I secured last week a large quantity of Podophyllum at 8¢ per pound. The price charged for this on former purchasing from a house in this city was 20¢.[141]

Another of Maisch's attempts to procure a direct supply of a native product occurred in 1862, before the laboratory began operations, when he encouraged American wine producers, especially in Ohio, to save the deposits in their wine casks for pharmaceutical and commercial uses.[142] This interest in American tartar was first of all due to Maisch's distrust of imported cream of tartar. Before the war he conducted analyses which indicated that the commercial product then on the market contained as much as 13 percent of tartrate of lime, and that it was adulterated with sand, gypsum, flour, chalk, alum, and potassium sulfate.[143] A second, but probably less significant reason for Maisch's concern, was the rising price of the red and white argols that were imported during the war. Mildew and vine rot destroyed much of the 1862 grape harvest,[144] but in 1863, with the permission of Andrew K. Smith, Maisch again entered into correspondence with the Wine Grower's Association in Ohio. Once again, however, his efforts failed to bring forward any substantial amount of crude tartar. Some tartar appeared on the market in Cincinnati, but only small quantities of it. Most of the wine makers sold their wines without keeping them for any length of time. Others who did age the wine were convinced that their stock was better kept in old casks with the tartar left in them.[145]

Testing to assure that crude drugs and finished pharmaceuticals met acceptable standards was one of the most important objectives that Hammond had in mind when he instituted the laboratories. Conferring with Andrew K. Smith after the Philadelphia laboratory had been operating only a few months, he decided that the time had come to direct Purveyor Murray to make no more purchases of drugs or liquors if specimens of them had not been tested at the laboratory.[146] Thereafter, testing operations became an increasingly significant part of Maisch's activities. Murray reserved the right to be guided in his decisions to purchase spirits by other evidence than the laboratory's reports— for example, by the knowledgeable taste of whiskey connoisseurs. Yet he sent samples of whiskey and brandy from reliable dealers to the laboratory for analysis before making his purchases.[147]

After the whiskey was bought and delivered to the laboratory, Maisch assayed samples taken from a few barrels in each lot to determine whether or not, within reasonable limits, they compared favorably with the original sample tested before the transaction.[148]

Not all the whiskey bottled at the laboratory went through tests before it arrived there. In one emergency, a shipment procured in Louisville by Medical Purveyor Meylert of that city was prepared for issue without the usual assays in Maisch's laboratory. Meylert had instead sent samples of the liquor to members of Hammond's staff in Washington, D.C. After tasting it, those in the surgeon general's office agreed that it was excellent whiskey. Such exceptions aside, Maisch's tests were as discriminating as the techniques of the times would permit. In addition to checking the specific gravity with an alcoholometer, Maisch used simple chemical reagents to discover impurities and adulterations, and Molnar's olfactory test to detect "the fusel oils of different origin."[149] In analyzing whiskey, Maisch declared his competence to apply Molnar's test, but he freely admitted that he lacked the experience to accurately distinguish the numerous varieties of brandy. With equal candor he acknowledged limitations of analytical chemistry which then existed by admitting that "precise chemical reactions would be of greater value" than the Molnar test.[150] Between October 1864 and the end of the war, Maisch tested sixty-seven samples of sherry wine for specific gravity, the percentage of alcohol, the volatile (acetic) acid, free tartaric acid, sugar, and "the extractive." Afterward he compiled a statistical chart from his data.[151]

From his earliest days in pharmacy, Maisch was always keenly aware of adulterations. When he was a clerk with Robert Shoemaker & Co. in the 1850s, he examined every consignment of drugs that came into their pharmacy, and not from idle curiosity, either, for at least one chemical manufacturer was surprised to find that some potassium iodide was returned from Shoemaker's because it did not come up to Maisch's requirements.[152] When he had been a member of the American Pharmaceutical Association for only a short time, Maisch became chairman of its important committee on adulterations and led in spirited discussions of the menace at the annual meetings. It was just as strongly characteristic of Maisch, however, that he should hold onto what was apparently a lifelong belief that close bargaining over the price of drugs was worse than useless. He was certain that willingness to pay a full price would invariably bring forth prime quality drugs, even in wartime.[153]

Because Maisch instructed Harrison Smith to buy nothing but the best in raw drugs and chemicals, relatively few of them arrived at the laboratory in an adulterated condition.[154] The drug dealers knew that Maisch would not only carefully scrutinize every item purchased, but also might publicize any adulterations by displaying them to the American Pharmaceutical Association, as he did a sample of benzoin in 1863, which he scornfully said was "chips of wood agglutinated by some gummy substance, containing not a trace of Benzoic acid, and but a slight trace of Cinnamic acid." Once or twice he rejected colchicum that was moldy, and on another occasion "some article resembling shoe-makers' wax, probably . . . black rosin, put up in rosin barrels and sent instead of it."[155] When he discovered that a shipment of lard contained from 10 percent to 12.5 percent water, which was held in suspension by potassium carbonate or borax, he refused to accept it.[156] In one cake of opium he discovered sixteen lead bullets. One medium-size bale of buchu leaves contained a stone weighing about ten pounds. He believed that "some terebinthi-nate oleoresin" was an adulterant in copaiba. In revelations of such adulterations, however, Maisch displayed little hostility to-ward the drug purveyors. At least he was not as critical as was Squibb.[157]

It is a singular fact that neither at Philadelphia nor at Astoria did the United States Army Laboratories manufacture as much as one ounce of quinine sulfate during the entire war. This was not, of course, because of any underestimation of the drug's impor-tance. As a febrifuge, and as a prophylactic against malaria, massive quantities of it were constantly in demand. Beginning with McClellan's peninsular campaign in 1862, it became a prac-tice to administer quinine to the officers and men "in whiskey in the early morning with or without coffee."[158] As one of the few drugs of that day having a rather dramatic specific effect, cinchona in its various forms had the reputation of a "wonder drug." It was prescribed not only for fever but also for scrofulous inflammation, rheumatism, neuralgia, dyspepsia, diarrhea, and venereal disease. Its tonic properties were universally acclaimed, and it was also used as an antiseptic, an astringent, a gargle, and even as a dentifrice.[159] From 1820 on, after the French pharmacists Pierre J. Pelletier and Joseph B. Caventou had isolated quinia and cinchonia (in the nomenclature of that day),[160] the preparation of quinine sulfate became a well-known and relatively simple pharmaceutical process. The chemist boiled the bark with muriatic acid, and treated the soluble muriate thus produced with lime to precipitate the quinine, after which he digested it in boiling alcohol to separate it from impurities and bleached it with boneblack.[161] It was therefore neither the unimportance of quinine nor technical problems in production that deterred the laboratories from manufacturing it.

Market conditions also seemed to indicate that the government would gain from manufacturing its own quinine. Only two American firms—Powers & Weightman and Rosengarten and Sons—produced it in quantity. In years with "sickly" autumns, the price underwent "a rapid and enormous rise" largely attributed to speculators trading in the drug market, especially in the South and in the fever-stricken Mississippi Valley, where[162] "P & W in bottles" was often the only quinine for sale.[163] Protected during the war by a 45 percent duty, quinine sulfate became most subject to speculation of all the drugs on the market. From a quotation of $2.10 an ounce in April 1861, it increased with violent fluctuations to $3.60 in May 1863.[164]

Hammond probably was more concerned about the high price of quinine than he was about any other pharmaceutical preparation on the supply table. During the weeks that immediately preceded the first operations at the Philadelphia laboratory, he was inquiring of the Philadelphia purveyor about the "feasibility of undertaking the manufacture of sulphate of quinine at the Laboratory."[165] On March 28, 1863, the surgeon general advised Satterlee, the New York City purveyor, to limit his purchases of quinine to no more than was absolutely required for current use, because "manufacture of the article" was "contemplated at the Laboratory in Philadelphia."[166] The manufacturers of quinine also became greatly interested, and deeply concerned, over the coming production of quinine at the laboratory. Andrew K. Smith confided to Hammond, "The manufacturing chemists here [Philadelphia] are in a great stew about our laboratory. Especially as they know that I am trying to estimate the cost of manufacturing quinine. Their squirming shows that their profits have been enormous."[167] In New York City, items published in the press indicated that the government's decision to manufacture its own quinine sulfate already had made a considerable impression on the drug market. *The New York Times* observed,

> The day after the publication in the *Times* of the intention of the Medical Department to manufacture its own quinine, the price of that article declined 33 per cent., and within a day or two past the Department has received propositions from parties in New York [City] and Philadelphia, offering to furnish the drug at a reduction of 70 cents per ounce. Speculators in the article have lost heavily.[168]

By the end of the war, the Philadelphia laboratory issued 23,088 ounces of powdered calisaya bark, 148,728 ounces of fluid extract of cinchonia with aromatics, 75,056 dozen quinine sulfate pills, and 9,790 ounces of citrate of iron and quinine. But neither at Philadelphia nor at Astoria was there manufactured one ounce of quinine sulfate or cinchona sulfate.

The reasons why this was not done have remained obscure. No evidence has turned up that Hammond, and after him, Barnes, had any clandestine arrangements with Powers & Weightman and the Rosengarten firm.[169] A possible motive that came out in the Hammond trial was the Medical Department's unwillingness to weaken the private American producers in the event foreign supplies of the drug should be shut off. At least, in April 1868, Hammond authorized Murray to purchase quinine sulfate from Rosengarten with the English price as a basis plus transportation, import duties, insurance, and exchange.[170] During the Hammond trial, when Murray testified on this order, he was asked the following question by the defense:

> Can you state whether or not the object of that authority was to encourage the manufacture of quinine in this country, so that in case of a difficulty in importation, we might have that manufactory here?[171]

Judge Advocate-General Holt did not permit Murray to answer the question, but the question may well have indicated Hammond's policy. Hammond also may have intended to use possible manufacture at the laboratory merely as a threat to hold down prices. A *New York Times* article documented the temporary success of this strategem. There was, however, another motivation of fundamental importance, directly related to the laboratory, namely that it would not be economical for the government to manufacture it there in view of the restricted supply of cinchona bark.

Hammond, at the outset of the laboratory project, informed Murray and Andrew K. Smith that the government would manufacture at the Philadelphia laboratory "whatever drugs and preparations for the use of this Dept. *you* shall deem [it] *economical* to manufacture."[172] Whatever his motive may have been, Smith directed Maisch, at Hammond's request, to prepare a statement on the economic feasibility of manufacturing quinine. In a long report, dated April 17, 1863, Maisch analyzed the problem with all his accustomed thoroughness and concluded that from an economic standpoint there was "very little probability . . . of preparing sulphate of quinia advantageously" at the laboratory.

His principal reasons for this conclusion all concerned the supply of cinchona bark, or more specifically (1) "that a constant supply of uniformly good Carthagena bark cannot be depended on"; (2) "the trade in these barks is chiefly in the hand of the quinia manufacturers"; and (3) "the government would probably have to pay the parties holding such bark a price high enough to exceed the actual market value of the quinia which is contained in it." Maisch's other reasons for discouraging the preparation of quinine sulfate at the laboratory were less important. They were the cost of new equipment needed for the operation, and that perhaps a new building would have to be procured for it.[173] Maisch went on to suggest that the laboratory should experiment in the manufacture of quinine sulfate. Bark was later ordered for these tests,[174] but they did not reverse Maisch's opinion against producing quinine sulfate at the laboratory.

If the Medical Department had been unable to resort to other expedients to meet its quinine problem the drug almost certainly would have been manufactured in Philadelphia. The department requisitioned some quinine (as well as other drugs) from the cargoes of prize vessels brought into American ports,[175] and it imported quinine from the British Isles upon which the Treasury Department remitted import duties.[176] The medical purveyors bought unbleached quinine (also known as hospital quinine) for about one-third less than they paid for the bleached product.[177] Finally, Hammond ordered cinchonia sulfate to be added to the supply table as an acceptable substitute for quinine sulfate.[178] At the time, five alkaloids of cinchona had been isolated sufficiently to be identified. In the nomenclature of that day they were quinia, quinidia, chinoidine, cinchonidia, and cinchonia. Beyond their empirical formulas little was known of them. Justus Liebig (1838) and A. Laurent (1841) reported the molecular formulas of quinia and cinchonia, and between 1880 and 1894, W. Königs, Z. Skraup, W. Miller, and Rhode worked out their constitution.[179] Cinchonia, chinoidine, and quinidia had been introduced as substitutes for quinia before the war but had not become popular drugs.[180]

Because it was a residual salt that remained in the "mother liquor" after quinia and quinidia had crystallized, cinchonia had accumulated in the possession of the manufacturers. Compared to quinine it had been overlooked, and even in 1863 sold for as little as forty-two cents per pound. When the supply table went through its revision in 1862, Hammond added it to the list. The manufacturers were then able to dispose of their supplies of it at a considerable profit, but doubtless it tended to hold down the price of quinine sulfate.[181] Late in the war there was still a large supply of cinchonia sulfate available, although it too began to rise in price.[182] From a theoretical viewpoint, cinchonia sulfate seemed to win quick acceptance. The apothecary of the Pennsylvania Hospital declared that the three cinchona alkaloids (quinidia, quinia, and cinchonia) were "used indiscriminately and in the same doses" in that hospital.[183] In India, three medical commissions appointed to assess the effectiveness of the cinchona alkaloids discovered that a mixture of the three alkaloids provided a drug just as effective as quinine sulfate, and "poor man's quinine" came into being.[184] The Madras Commission's analysts, however, found cinchonia to be considerably inferior to the other alkaloids.[185] During the Civil War, some physicians insisted that larger doses of it were necessary to get comparable results, and that it was "more variable and less reliable than the quinia salt."[186] Cinchonia sulfate was officinal in the fourth revision of the United States Pharmacopoeia,[187] although quinidia sulfate—which Pepper and other outstanding practitioners prescribed in the same or smaller doses than quinine sulfate[188]— was not.

The persisting muddiness of the cinchona problem and policy reflected partly the indecisive scientific means then available to evaluate the alkaloids therapeutically. But, more broadly, it reflected partly the indecisive social means to evaluate when the government could or should intrude into a private sanctum, such as the small, closed world of the cinchona and quinine market. At best the government laboratories must have been considered an unwelcome experiment by private pharmaceutical manufacturers. At least the main part of the business community probably considered it an unjustified experiment. As for the Medical Department, there is no evidence that Surgeon General Barnes, or even Hammond, ever considered the laboratories more than a temporary expedient that could be of little, if any, service to the government after the war.

Chapter 5

The Balance Sheet

Demobilization of the Union armies began almost as soon as the guns fell silent. Less than three weeks after Lee's surrender at Appomattox, General Orders No. 77 directed that bureau heads in the War Department should reduce "the number of . . . employees to that [number] absolutely required for closing the business of their respective departments."[1] The surgeon general in particular received instructions to make drastic reductions in the Medical Department's staff.[2] At the beginning of May, Andrew K. Smith complied by reducing his working force in the sewing department by 25 percent and the employees in the chemical department "to the lowest amount of force consistent with the requirements of the service."[3] There was, however, no immediate order to terminate activities at the laboratories.

It is understandable that Joseph H. Bill and Andrew K. Smith, who had put forth so much effort in building up their laboratories, would be loath to see them shut down. In his report of December 31, 1864, before the fire at Astoria, Bill proposed that a permanent laboratory in the vicinity of New York City might continue to give the Medical Department financial savings after the war. He wrote:

> It is suggested that it would be well worth-while to establish a Laboratory permanently but on a legal and legislative basis. If the miserable collection of sheds at this place affording only half the supplies for the medical department

can save over four hundred thousand dollars per annum . . . surely a well-appointed laboratory on a selected site, well-designed and built could do much better. . . . An establishment such as I have indicated with the apparatus now on hand furnishing supplies for the whole army could be built exclusive of land for one hundred thousand dollars and be a credit to the department and government. If made too large for times of peace the surplus room could be used as a purveying Depot. My estimate made at present prices and the plan I have drawn is for a two-story brick building having an area on the ground floor of fifty thousand square feet besides outbuildings covering fifteen thousand feet more . . .[4]

Surgeon General Barnes not only refused to give any consideration to this plan, he even rejected any proposal to restore the Astoria laboratory after its fire in February 1865. As the period of liquidation began, however, the resourceful Andrew K. Smith, although he did not make any proposal like Bill's for a postwar laboratory, attempted to keep his personnel together and to stretch out the operations of the Philadelphia laboratory as long as possible. In June 1865, the surgeon general's office apparently gave brief consideration to a proposal of Medical Purveyor McDougall that the ether-making facilities at the laboratory should continue to produce that anesthetic for the entire army.[5] The suggestion was not accepted, but a decision was made that month to the effect that after reducing expenses to "the lowest practicable point," articles would continue to be manufactured there "from time to time . . . for present use."[6]

Huge surplus stocks of medical supplies in the various purveying depots' warehouses presented another problem, especially in New York City and Philadelphia, where they were especially large. Satterlee was quite pleased with himself for a clever negotiation by which he induced the navy to accept many of these articles at a price that the navy officials soon regretted,[7] but there were also auction sales to dispose of a long list of medicines and hospital supplies.[8] A large public sale took place in Philadelphia on August 4th.[9] Throughout the autumn and winter months, even into the spring of 1866, Purveyor McDougall continued to make private contracts for such items as metallic bismuth, lard ("slightly rancid"), potash, ground flaxseed, belladonna leaves, buchu, mustard, gamboge, calisaya bark, Jamaica ginger, "blue mass," mercurial ointment, ipecac, ether, and other drugs.[10] Comparing the prices received for them with the prevailing quotations on the New York City wholesale market, the contracts made for the surplus items were either the equivalent or only slightly less than those on the drug exchange. Andrew K. Smith with his usual perspicacity also tried to induce the surgeon general's office to give the Philadelphia laboratory an additional function—to serve as a center, at least in the East, for the preparation for sale of drugs from most of the purveying depots.[11] In the surgeon general's words, "a vast amount" of medicines and hospital supplies were collected at Philadelphia and other "prominent points" for disposal at public auction,[12] but by November 1865, the Astoria laboratory was at an end.

Bill had so little to do there that he received orders to relieve the medical storekeeper at the New York City purveying depot on such occasions as Satterlee might direct him.[13] Bids were taken for the equipment at Astoria purveying depot, and after some delays caused by the slowness of the auctioneers, the public property finally was disposed of there in December.[14] At the Philadelphia laboratory, meanwhile, two of Smith's able hospital stewards were mustered out of the service on August 1.[15] Near the end of October there arrived from the surgeon general's office positive orders to "dispense with the services" of Maisch not later than November 1 and, "taking into consideration the large amount of supplies now on hand," to reduce other expenses to a bare minimum required to supply an army of 100,000 men.[16]

The next to leave the Philadelphia laboratory after Maisch was Andrew K. Smith who, late in November, was transferred to the Department of South Carolina, where he became medical director. His successor at Philadelphia was none other than Joseph H. Bill, who probably brought with him, ironically enough, a small amount of equipment that he salvaged from the Astoria laboratory before the auctions.[17]

Bill became director of the Philadelphia laboratory around January 1, 1866, and remained there, supervising the bottling of liquors and carrying on pharmaceutical manufacturing operations, including some quinine products, for twenty-nine months. His workforce, compared to the war years, was a very small crew—two clerks, four laborers, and four watchmen—and his payroll was but $500 per month.[18] Their main task was to produce for issue the bulk drugs that were at the laboratory or brought into it from other depots.[19] By November 1867, preparations were being made to sell the laboratory apparatus and to close the establishment, but because the money market was very tight, the sale of the apparatus was delayed until January 15, 1868.[20] On February 18, one of Bill's last shipments—10,000 bottles of whiskey—was ready for transportation, although he apparently continued his bottling operations into March 1868.[21] But at the end of April, Bill notified the surgeon general that except for the completion of his accounts (which he would do quickly), the business of the laboratory was finished. He requested reassignment to the Department of Columbia in the Pacific Northwest. Special Orders No. 110 sent him to Fort Vancouver and on May 20 he retired from his duties at the laboratory.[22] The only remaining responsibility was for McDougall to turn over the laboratory's records to the post's quartermaster for transportation to the surgeon general's office.[23]

The success or failure, achievements and shortcomings of the laboratories may be partially evaluated by briefly reviewing their records against the anticipated advantages that Surgeon General

Barnes outlined in September 1863. These briefly stated were
(1) "the securing of perfect purity in our drugs and chemicals,"
(2) "the saving to the Government of the profits now secured by
the parties furnishing drugs etc.," (3) "perfect uniformity in the
mode of putting up our supplies," (4) "to ascertain beforehand
the purity or impurity of crude drugs and liquors and hospital
stores offered for sale," i.e., the testing of bulk drugs, liquors, etc.
at the laboratories, and (5) to "control the prices of the articles
manufactured."[24]

The laboratory directors, John Maisch, and other personnel all
took great pride in the quality of the medical supplies that came
out of the laboratories. The existing records and correspondence
agree with Bill's assertion[25] that there were few complaints from
the armies in the field or from the hospitals against the quality of
the laboratory products. There was, in fact, only one known
protest against a product from the Astoria laboratory, lodged by a
surgeon in the Army of the James who claimed that powdered
acacia that bore the laboratory's seal was "unfit for use as medicine." It was, ironically, Charles McCormick, at the time he was
medical director of the department and purveyor at Norfolk, who
answered the charge while in the field near Bermuda Hundred.
He conceded that the acacia was adulterated, although not with
"pepper or some other acrid substance," but rather was contami-
nated with *Calamus aromaticus.*[26]

Chloroform was one of the few products criticized by users of
preparations manufactured at the Philadelphia laboratory. Following major engagements when there was for several days a
shortage of that anesthetic on the battlefield, Maisch admitted
that the standards of inspection were lowered, as orders flooded
the laboratory. Presumably quality was sacrificed to some degree
on such occasions. In describing one such emergency, Maisch
wrote:

Immediately after the battle of Gettysburg a large quantity
of Chloroform then on hand at the Laboratory for purification, had to be put up for the emergency, because the market
was completely exhausted of pure Chloroform. Since there
was not time enough allowed then to have different labels
printed, we endeavored to buy labels without the Laboratory mark upon them but failing this we were compelled to
use our own. Some of the Chloroform may have remained
on hand and cannot now be distinguished from that of our
own manufacture.[27]

The most serious criticism of the Philadelphia laboratory's
chloroform came after the war's last battle had been fought. On
May 22, 1865, Barnes ordered McDougall to send to his office
one pound of chloroform in a glass-stoppered bottle and an equal
amount in a metal container, both samples to be as they were
prepared in the laboratory.[28] Over two months later, Joseph J.
Woodward of the surgeon general's office transmitted a report of
assistant surgeon B. F. Craig, which declared that a sample of
chloroform from the laboratory was "impure."[29] From the subse-
quent correspondence it can be inferred that the supposed impurities resulted from decomposition, with resulting liberation of
chlorine and hydrochloric acid. Even before this report the laboratory had received a preliminary condemnation of the chloroform and instructions to "issue no more chloroform from the
laboratory at Philadelphia until the entire amount on hand . . .
[could] be reexamined and purified."[30]

Maisch then entered into an exchange of correspondence with
Craig, through Director Smith, and at the same time began a
thorough examination of possible causes for the impurities. In
his first response to the charges, Maisch denied that methyl alcohol had been used in preparation of chloroform at the laboratory
(thus refuting one of the specific allegations in Craig's report).
He admitted, however, that the hospital steward who had been in

charge of the chloroform still had changed the sulfuric acid used in the purification process but once in five months, and that particularly in busy times—as during the weeks that followed the Astoria fire when he was working until eleven or twelve o'clock each night—he was obliged to "leave the easy tests to the assistants of the various departments." He recalled also that he had on occasion returned several hundred bottles of chloroform to the filling department for rerectification.[31]

After receiving the complaint lodged by Woodward, Maisch personally opened and examined nearly all of the chloroform in the laboratory's storeroom and at the Philadelphia purveying depot, and submitted it to further purification.[32] In the course of his examination, Maisch discovered that the laboratory's chloroform did indeed decompose more rapidly than that of other manufacturers. He also found out that the reason for it was the higher specific gravity of the laboratory's product, and the fact that it was exposed to light. His practical conclusion was that, to "keep it from getting acid," the chloroform should be reduced in specific gravity to about 1.475 by the addition of alcohol.[33] This was, indeed, something that Squibb already had learned during the war when his chloroform had undergone similar decomposition as it was jostled during transportation to the battlefields.[34] It was later verified to a certain degree by Schnacht, Blitz, and Brown, who concluded that, although chloroform was not decomposed in the absence of oxygen by sunlight, the addition of alcohol, one part in 400, was "sufficient to prevent recognizable decomposition for one month or longer," and double that amount of alcohol would prevent it for a year.[35]

The only other question known to have been raised about the quality of the Philadelphia laboratory's products, and it was not as challenging as the chloroform question, concerned isinglass plaster. In this case, Thomas Antisell[36] reported (May 15, 1864) that the ichthyocolla plaster was "worthless because if [sic] its imperfect and unequal mode of spreading and its surface not having the proper varnish coating."[37] Andrew K. Smith then explained that the plaster that brought forth the complaint was "the tail end of a piece of silk stretched upon the machine," a remnant such as the employees were instructed never to package.[38] Not being content merely to answer the charge, Smith then secured testimonials on the quality of the laboratory's plasters from surgeons and hospital administrators.[39] In one of these, John L. LeConte, the medical inspector at Philadelphia, declared that he had never heard any complaints against them.[40]

One other conflict over purity of drugs developed when Maisch tried to ensure greater purity of medicinal spirits—Spiritus Lavandulae Compositus and Spiritus Ammoniae Aromaticus—which were on the supply table and were produced in sizeable quantities at the laboratory. This lively controversy did not concern the surgeon general's office directly, but rather Edward R. Squibb and other leaders of the American Pharmaceutical Association. It began when Maisch, with the consent of Andrew K. Smith, ordered that with the exception of the oil of lemon used in the Spiritus Ammoniae Aromaticus, both of the medicinal spirits should be made from distillation of the crude drugs rather than using their essential oils as the United States Pharmacopoeia directed. Maisch believed that there were sufficient reasons for the change, because lavender flowers, rosemary leaves, and the other constituents would be pure and less expensive than the frequently adulterated oils. He proudly brought samples of both preparations of his manufacture to the American Pharmaceutical Association meeting in 1864, and in a volunteer paper reported that numerous army surgeons had declared their satisfaction with the spirits made by the Maisch formula.[41]

It was obvious that Maisch not only hoped but believed that his alteration in the Pharmacopoeia's directions would be adopted by the committee on revision and incorporated in the fifth decennial revision (1870).[42] Instead, he unexpectedly found himself censured by Squibb and Ferdinand F. Mayer (the Committee on

Volunteer Papers), who reported to the executive committee that they acted not because of Maisch's "fair and legitimate criticism upon officinal medicated waters and spirits" or his offer of "improved formulas," but because he was adopting such formulas at the laboratory and implying that they were preferred to officinal formulas in army medical practice.[43] Such practices, Squibb argued, could only weaken the prestige of the Pharmacopoeia.[44]

The Maisch-Squibb debate continued at the association's meeting in 1865, when Maisch, in a counterattack, accused Squibb of similarly departing from the Pharmacopoeia's formula by substituting resin of scammony for scammony in compound extract of colocynth.[45] Parrish also entered the argument on the side of his friend, Maisch, when he asserted that Squibb was too strict in his construction of the Pharmacopoeia's meaning. Being aware that Maisch's controversial formula for Spiritus Lavandulae Compositus made forty gallons of the distillate in one operation,[46] Parrish observed:

> Everybody must use his judgment, and interpret the Pharmacopoeia according to common sense. Suppose, instead of preparing a pint of fluid extract, as ordered by the Pharmacopoeia, I make ten gallons. I maintain that this is an entirely different thing. Adhere to the spirit of the Pharmacopoeia; it is not necessary to adhere to the letter.[47]

In this statement Parrish hit upon an important fact imperfectly recognized at the time, that new developments in industrial pharmacy, typified by operations at the United States Army Laboratories, were revealing practical limitations of a pharmacopoeia that described formulas designed for use in small pharmacies. Diehl, for example, in making collodion at the Philadelphia laboratory, discovered that in immersing cotton in a solution of potassium nitrate and sulfuric acid for twenty-four hours the temperature required for the solution in the Pharmacopoeia might be suitable for quantities measured in ounces, but "totally beyond control when applied to a manufacturing scale."[48] Maisch similarly advised Andrew K. Smith: "It is obvious that the scale on which we manufacture requires a departure from the minutiae laid down in the directions of the Pharmacopoeia, which are intended for operations on a small scale only. . . ."[49]

The fact that Maisch had touched a broadening need of the future became obvious in the first decade of the twentieth century, when Joseph P. Remington tried to answer a question concerning the eighth revision of the Pharmacopoeia. The question was: "Is it true that the United States Pharmacopoeia (8th revision) is more of a Manufacturer's Handbook than a Pharmacist's Guide?" Remington's answer was significant. It demonstrated the distance pharmacy had traveled since the Maisch-Squibb debate of 1865, as Remington explained:

> It [the Pharmacopoeia] is certainly to be considered a manufacturer's hand-book because there is no doubt that the pharmacist of today sells more products manufactured by others, than he does preparations made by himself; and it is a pharmacist's guide, because, by its use, the pharmacist is enabled to keep the manufacturer's goods up to standard.[50]

The second of Barnes' "anticipated advantages" at the laboratories, the savings which the government could make by eliminating the profits of private drug manufacturers, is more controversial than the purity of the laboratories' products. With the exception of a few critics in the surgeon general's office, no one has ever challenged the competence or fidelity of the men who administered the laboratories. The few commentaries that have been written upon the laboratories have all agreed that they saved the government large sums of money during the war by providing medical supplies at a cost lower than the market prices.

Every laboratory administrator, Bill, Smith, Maisch, and even Creamer at St. Louis cited figures to prove that these savings were real. As early as September 1863, for example, Andrew K.

Smith was comparing in one of his reports the lower "cost of the Articles as made" at the laboratory as compared with the "price list of prominent houses." Simple cerate, he asserted, cost the laboratory (including tinned cans, labeling, and "putting up") thirty-seven cents per pound, compared to the Hance, Griffith & Co.'s quotation of 50 cents. Powders at the laboratory were manufactured at 60 percent less than the commercial firms were selling them for. Precipitated chalk cost the laboratory eight cents per pound, but that of Powers and Weightman could be bought for no less than eighteen cents. Blue pill mass was made at the laboratory for 37⅝ cents per pound but Squibb's price was 60 cents.[51] Comparisons of this kind carried throughout the entire list of products suggested impressive savings for the government, especially since its own costs did not take into account certain expenses normal to private competitive enterprise. Andrew K. Smith probably drew upon Maisch's statistics for his statements, as Maisch apparently kept a very careful record, taken directly from the laboratory's ledgers.

In compiling his statistics at Astoria, Bill arrived at the market price of items not normally listed on the drug exchange by requesting Squibb, Schieffelin and Brothers, and Philip Schieffelin & Co. (the three firms that Satterlee dealt with most often before the Astoria laboratory operated) "to state at what price per pound they would furnish such articles of the supply table." Then he took the average of the three quotations as his market value. Squibb was probably the most important source of information in establishing these figures. There is every indication that Bill also tried to establish accurately the cost of his laboratory's products. Besides the cost of raw materials and other such expense, he included operating expenses such as general labor, gas, fuel, and maintenance to arrive at an actual cost total.

The statistics for the Astoria laboratory, unfortunately, are incomplete, but for the six months ending November 30, 1864, Bill reported the savings to the government at $279,972.04.[52]

Maisch, who also compared the cost of the Philadelphia laboratory's products with the market price at the time they were issued, claimed the financial savings to the government were $766,019.32 from March 1863 to September 30, 1865.[53] Hammond was not quite as optimistic, but nevertheless agreed that the United States had saved nearly half a million dollars from the Philadelphia establishment.[54] Smith was most expansive of all, saying that the government's savings ran to a million dollars or more during the two years and eight months that he was superintendent of the laboratory.[55] Alfred Stillé, in a postwar account of Hammond's achievements which was quoted in a Senate Report, was less specific when he avowed that the laboratories saved the government "the outlay of large sums of money."[56] W. C. Spencer, writing the half page allotted to the history of the laboratories in the *Medical and Surgical History of the War of the Rebellion,* presented these quoted figures of Maisch and Bill.[57]

Granting the honesty and care with which Maisch and Bill assembled their data, there are four factors that cast doubt upon the savings which they claimed from the laboratories' operations.

First, the large amounts of medical supplies that were sold at public or private sale after the war went for prices close to or slightly below the wholesale market quotations of that day. But many of these supplies were manufactured during the war when costs of materials, labor, and so forth were considerably higher.

Second, the machinery was often run to the limit of its capacity as the working hours stretched out into overtime. As Bill admitted, the intensive effort was "expensive and wasteful, wearing out the machinery."[58] To be sure, Bill and Maisch evidently included maintenance and repairs in their costs, but there is no indication that they allowed for the rapid depreciation of their equipment.

Third, the sales of laboratory apparatus when the laboratories were finally liquidated were disappointing to the Medical Department. Powers & Weightman, for example, offered $4,000 for all the Philadelphia machinery, with only a few pieces excepted, but its original price had been $21,700. As McDougall put it, the bid hardly amounted to "the price of old copper" in the apparatus.[59] Largely because of the disastrous fire, but possibly also for other reasons, Bill's list of property lost by accident, which was filed at the close of the Astoria laboratory's operations, resulted in a request from the surgeon general for "a detailed statement of the circumstances that caused such a heavy loss of property."[60]

Fourth, and last, many of the laboratories' expenses were charged off to other departments of the federal government and not accounted for as their own costs. Bill considered all expenses for warming and heating his bottling department to be properly chargeable to the Quartermaster Department.[61] The same agency took care of the laboratories' drayage—both of raw materials and finished products. As has been noted, the quartermaster agreed to pay rent for the laboratory buildings.[62] Even the articles acquired free by Andrew K. Smith in his scavenging forays belonged to some other agency of the federal government. It is doubtful that the wages of the hospital stewards employed at the laboratories were charged to their account.

All these costs eventually had to be paid by the taxpayer, but they did not appear as expenses of the laboratories. This is not to say, however, that the laboratories did not achieve any savings. Barnes pointed out in September 1863 that the manufacturers' profits ranged from 12 to 33 percent.[63] At the end of the war, one of the pharmacist's own publications noted that for reliable products the manufacturers' markups always assured them of a 20 percent profit.[64] Operating efficiently, the laboratories were able to afford the government savings[65] compared to the wholesale prices.[66] The percentage of savings, however, was less than Maisch, Bill, and others claimed.

There is no question about Barnes' third expected advantage, if it is specifically considered. The methods of preparation varied somewhat from day to day, and from Astoria to Philadelphia, but there most certainly was "uniformity in preparation," including packaging and labeling. If, however, Barnes implied that he was expecting what apparently had been the goal of Andrew K. Smith at the outset of the laboratory program, namely, complete uniformity in the medical supplies of the Union army arising from the manufacture of everything needed at the laboratories,[67] such a goal was never attained. During the two years of the war in which they existed, the laboratories turned out varying percentages of the preparations on the standard supply table. In some instances their combined production approached a complete supply of the government's needs for a particular article, but of other items they turned out either small amounts or none at all. By the autumn of 1863 when, according to Barnes, the Philadelphia laboratory was still in a "limited and experimental" stage of operations,[68] there had been accumulated at the purveying depots sufficient medicines to supply three million men in the field for three months.[69] Most of the preparations on the supply table, except for dressings, chloroform, opium, and a few others, were stored in "great excess" at the warehouses for the remainder of the war.[70] It was seldom that the Philadelphia laboratory found itself hard pressed to meet current demands. It was with respect to chloroform after Gettysburg, and it was again in the spring of 1864, when some of its shipments lacked certain items (such as tartaric acid) and requisitions took all the opium that had been powdered and prepared at the laboratory.[71]

Not even Hammond attempted to make the laboratories the sole suppliers of the armies. During the summer of 1863, the Cincinnati purveyor received instructions to purchase many articles on his requisitions in Cincinnati to replenish his stocks as it was supposed "that the cost of transportation, packing etc. would more than cover the difference in the market price between Philadelphia and Cincinnati. . . ."[72] Again, Joseph R. Smith explained the Medical Department's procurement policy:

In regards to articles to be purchased in Louisville . . . this will be the principle governing in issuing instructions: Such articles as we can supply from our own laboratories in Phila. and N. Y. [City] will be sent you, and such articles as can undoubtedly be purchased and sent at less expense than you can buy. Other articles you will buy, and generally by contract it is expected . . .[73]

Most of the medicines at Mower Hospital and the other general hospitals in the vicinity of Philadelphia came from the laboratory in that city,[74] and the medical purveyor in Baltimore was also supplied largely from there. In May 1864, for example, Andrew K. Smith was asked if he could furnish the Baltimore purveyor with medicines for 50,000 men in the field and 20,000 more in general hospitals.[75] One of its most versatile operations came in the spring of 1865 when it filled more than seventy of the Autenrieth medicine wagons for the Army of the Potomac.[76] The Medical Department, however, continued to import manufactured drugs from abroad (it purchased them in bond without paying duties), and bought from wholesalers and manufacturers in Philadelphia and New York City. After the isinglass plaster incident, the surgeon general's office instructed Murray to purchase that preparation (although it was still being turned out at the Philadelphia laboratory) not only from Philadelphia supply houses, but also from those who offered it to the government in Camden.[77] In his explanation of how the laboratory shared with "private parties," the Medical Department's orders for supplies, Maisch wrote:

When the laboratory went into operation, the stock of medical supplies on hand at the purveying depot in this city was very large, some portions of it never being exhausted through the continuance of the war. . . . Moreover, preparations which were on hand, or to make which we possessed all the facilities, were frequently bought in the market or

ordered from private parties by medical purveyors in other
cities, so that we occasionally worked to replenish our stock
while such private parties worked for immediate supply.[78]

In summary, the laboratories did provide a uniformity to the
medical supplies that they issued, but side-by-side with their
uniform packages and labels there continued to be, as earlier in
the war, the various products of private manufacturers acquired
through commercial channels.

The United States Army Laboratories did not cause any no-
ticeable stagnation in the American pharmaceutical industry. Indeed the manufacturing processes in the laboratories paralleled
the development of privately owned enterprises, and the extraordinary demand for medicines during the war stimulated pharmaceutical manufacturing of all kinds, from the cheapest nos-
trums to the finest officinal products. As Evan Tyson Ellis
recalled many years after the war, "This was war-time, and trade
was very active; every old thing was salable in the way of
drugs."[79] George D. Rosengarten had an income of $98,526 in
1864, and William D. Weightman was not far behind him with
$83,255."[80] Even the drug mills prospered; one of them adver-
tised in 1865 that he had recently made large additions to his
machinery, and introduced several new improvements at his
works."[81]

It was during the war years and immediately thereafter that
interesting new business ventures appeared and the expansion of
older firms occurred. If Squibb, for example, failed to procure all
the government orders that he had anticipated early in the war, his
business nevertheless prospered, as he received more contracts
from the Medical Department for filling an improved type of
pannier.[82] Realizing that the Civil War was going to hasten the
transition from mortar and pestle to machine production, William
Henry Schieffelin and his associates built laboratory facilities, invented new apparatus, and improved their methods especially in

the manufacture of fluid extracts.[83] Edward Parrish formed a partnership to enlarge his production of the newly developing resinoids, extracts, and other drugs.[84] In Cincinnati, W. J. M. Gordon and Brother rapidly increased their output of glycerin and prepared to begin the extraction of bromine from the western salt brines.[85] Other pharmaceutical manufacturers began to compete with the British chemical exporters for the control of the American market with such articles as sodium carbonate and potassium iodide.[86] New mechanical means of counting and packaging pills made their appearance.[87] William Richard Warner founded a wholesale drug business in Philadelphia. Ten years later, he occupied a six-story building.[88] From the 1860 census figures to those of the ninth census (1870), the number of establishments in the United States manufacturing medicines, extracts, and drugs increased from 173 to 292 establishments, the number employed from 1,059 to 4,729 persons, and the capital invested from $1,977,385 to $12,750,809.[89]

Barnes' fourth reason for viewing the laboratories optimistically was that they would have "facilities for correct analysis of all articles liable to adulteration previous to purchase." These assays were carried on more intensively by Maisch at Philadelphia than they were under Bill's direction at Astoria. This is not to say that Bill minimized them, but for Maisch they were a major achievement. The testing program, however, did not proceed without a challenge from Joseph Janvier Woodward and his small staff who tested drugs, food extracts, and liquors in a laboratory associated directly with the surgeon general's office in Washington, D.C. At times Woodward tested simultaneously the raw drugs and spirits sent to the Philadelphia laboratory for assays, and he occasionally—for instance when an allotment of sherry wine had caused complaints—retested articles that had been given tests at the laboratory.[90] Correspondence on these testing procedures between Maisch and Woodward brought out strong differences of opinion with Woodward frequently criticizing Maisch's results.[91]

Woodward apparently was able to convince Barnes that the Philadelphia laboratory was using whiskey tests in some degree unsatisfactory, because Barnes, in the spring of 1864, requested A. D. Bache, President of the National Academy of Science, to consider what could be done to better detect adulterations in whiskey. A committee of the academy then recommended that Congress appropriate $43,500 to bring about the discovery of a "correct and practical test of the purity and medicinal value of whiskies."[92] Satterlee was later authorized to pay accounts presented for the necessary expenses (up to $3,500) incurred by the academy in carrying out the study.[93]

Maisch believed that his testing of crude drugs not only was a guarantee that the laboratory would produce pure medicines but also that he thereby exercised a beneficent influence upon the quality of goods imported into the United States. If a large purchaser such as the Medical Department rejected "every drug and preparation not of standard quality," others too would be more careful in their selection of raw drugs. Eventually, foreign dealers would experience a demand for their best offerings. In 1864, Maisch thought that he saw a trend in that direction.[94] It is impossible to say whether or not he was correct in his assumptions. It would be possible to argue that the purchases of the government buyers in the market often took up the most desirable grades of a crude drug and forced others to accept what was left, or that in its great need, as in the case of quinine, the government took up nearly everything available.[95]

The same question might be asked with respect to the fifth advantage that Barnes claimed for the laboratories, namely, that they could "control the prices of articles manufactured." There can be little doubt that the operations of the laboratories had a psychological influence on the drug market. As late as January 1864, for example, one writer familiar with pharmaceutical sales still believed that the laboratories were largely supplying the armies with quinine.[96] As a yardstick against which to measure the prices and quality of the commercial producers' articles the laboratories were always significant, for what they manufactured and even more for what they might produce if the government could not buy on satisfactory terms. As the pharmaceutical industry expanded during the war, the supply of some drugs became more regularized, and speculative operations—which had fed on the uncertainty of foreign goods arriving—began to slacken, even though prices, compared to antebellum days, remained high.[97] But medicines, like every other commodity, continued to move up and down with the price of gold, tariff duties, the course of the war, and other extraneous factors. Just what influence, if any, the laboratories had upon prices among all the other factors remains a matter of conjecture.

The United States Army Laboratories may not have achieved all the goals that Hammond envisioned for them or that Barnes accepted as advantages in their operations. But all four of the army officers who played principal roles in their administration received brevets for "faithful and meritorious service." Smith was a brevet lieutenant colonel (March 13, 1865); Satterlee became a brevet brigadier general (the rank which he had so long coveted); Murray, brevet colonel, March 13, 1865 (to become surgeon general in 1883); and Bill, brevet lieutenant colonel, March 13, 1865.[98]

For all of his brilliant services, John M. Maisch received no public citation from his government. He was a German immigrant, a member of a profession that medical men were wont to "handle without gloves,"[99] and a civilian employee of an Army Medical Department that had learned much from the experiences of the war but still was dominated by snobbish cliques. He had testified at the trial of the imaginative and dynamic creator of the laboratories only to see him cashiered.

Perhaps because they owed their existence to Hammond, the laboratories were to receive little recognition for their contributions to the Union's cause.[100] A lone suggestion in the *Army and Navy Journal* that they might be continued to provide a training school for pharmacists who would form a corps of apothecaries in the army after the war fell on deaf ears.[101] And when the surgeon general's office began to collect materials for the *Medical and Surgical History of the War of the Rebellion,* Procter's request that the story of the laboratories should be fully told therein was all but ignored.[102] Two short paragraphs from a report by W. C. Spencer was the extent of coverage in that work.[103] For a time, Procter believed that the War Department was even reluctant to release for publication statistics or other information on the operations of the laboratories.[104] But when Maisch left the Philadelphia laboratory for the last time in November 1865, to open a small pharmacy on Ridge Avenue, he asked for no plaudits from generals or politicians. His fame was secure as one of the greatest American pharmacists.

Appendix A

Materia Medica and Preparations on the U.S. Army Supply Table During the Civil War, Together with Constituent Drugs and Chemicals

Acaciae Pulvis
"The concrete juice of Acacia Vera and other species of acacia"*
Powdered (USP, 4th rev., p. 9).
Acidum Aceticum
Crude acetic acid produced by destructive distillation of wood
Cream of lime (calx)
Sulfuric acid
Sodium sulfate
Sodium sulfate
Sodium chloride
Sulfuric acid

Directions Concerning the Manner of Obtaining and Accounting for Medical and Hospital Supplies for the Army with a Standard Supply Table (Washington, Government Printing Office, 1862), pp. 7-9.

Water is not always indicated as a constituent. Data is from the following: *The Pharmacopoeia of the United States* (Fourth Decennial Revision, Philadelphia, J. B. Lippincott & Co., 1863), p. 399; George B. Wood and Franklin Bache, *The Dispensatory of the United States of America* (Eleventh and Twelfth Editions, Philadelphia, J. B. Lippincott & Co., 1858, 1866); Edward Parrish, *A Treatise on Pharmacy* (Third Edition, Philadelphia, Blanchard and Lea, 1864), 850 pp.; Frederic John Farre et al. *Manual of Materia Medica & Therapeutics,* Horatio C. Wood Jr. ed. (Philadelphia, Henry C. Lea, 1866), 1030 pp.

*All or a major part of the supply was imported.

Acidum Citricum
   Lime or lemon juice*
   Chalk*
   Sulfuric acid
Acidum Muriaticum
   Sodium chloride
   Sulfuric acid
Acidum Nitricum
   Potassium nitrate* or Sodium nitrate*
   Sulfuric acid
Acidum Phosphoricum Dilutum
   Phosphorus*
   Nitric acid
   Distilled water
Acidum Sulphuricum
   Sulfur*
   Potassium nitrate* or Sodium nitrate*
Acidum Sulphuricum Aromaticum
   Sulfuric acid
   Cinnamon*
   Ginger*
Acidum Tannicum
   Powdered nutgalls*
   Ether
      Ether
         Stronger alcohol
         Sulfuric acid
         Potassium
         Distilled water
Acidum Tartaricum
   Sulfuric acid
   Tartar (argols)*
   Carbonate of lime
Aether Fortior
   Ether
   Calcium chloride
   Lime

Aetheris Spiritus Compositus (Hoffmann's Anodyne)
    Ether
    Alcohol
    Oleum Aethereum (Ethereal Oil)
        Oleum Aethereum
            Stronger ether
            Stronger alcohol
            Sulfuric acid
            Distilled water
Aetheris Spiritus Nitrici
    Nitric acid
    Stronger alcohol
    Potassium carbonate
Alcohol Fortius
    Rectified spirit
    Potassium carbonate
Aloes Pulvis (Aloes purificata)
    Socotrine aloes* (other varieties also used)
    Stronger alcohol
Alumen (Potassium Alum)*
    "Sulphate of alumina and potassa" or alum ore* (USP, 4th rev.,
    p. 15). (*Note:* Ammonium Alum was officinal in USP, 4th rev.,
    p. 15, and it was manufactured by Powers & Weightman from
    the liquor of gas works, but it was not listed on the supply table.)
Ammoniae Carbonas (Ammonium carbonate)
    Sal ammoniac*
    Chalk*
Ammoniae Liquor
    Solution of ammonia
    Distilled water
        Ammonia
            Sal ammoniac*
            Dry quicklime
Ammoniae Murias (Sal ammoniac)*
    Derived from liquor of gas works
Ammoniae Spiritus Aromaticus
    Ammonium carbonate
    Ammonia water

Oil of lemon*
Oil of nutmeg*
Oil of lavender*
Alcohol
Antimonii et Potassae Tartratis Pulvis (Tartar emetic)[†]
    Oxide of antimony*
    Purified tartar*
    Distilled water
Argenti Nitras
    Silver
    Nitric acid
    Distilled water
Argenti Nitras Fusus
    Silver nitrate
    Muriatic acid
Arsenitis Potassae Liquor
    Arsenious acid*
    Potassium bicarbonate (saleratus)*
    Compound spirit of lavender
    Distilled water
Assafoetida
    "The concrete juice of the root of Narthex Assafoetida"*
    (USP, 4th rev., p. 18).
Bismuthi Subcarbonas
    Bismuth*
    Nitric acid
    Ammonia water
    Carbonate of soda*
    Distilled water
Camphora
    "A peculiar concrete substance derived from Camphora
    officinarum"* (USP, 4th rev., p. 22).
    Purified by sublimation
Cantharidis Ceratum
    Cantharidis*
    Yellow wax (beeswax)

[†]This was omitted from the May 7, 1863 revision of the standard supply table.

Resin
Lard
Cantharidis Pulvis
"Cantharis vesicatoria"* (USP, 4th rev., p. 22).
Capsici Pulvis
"The fruit of Capsicum annuum, and of other species of Capsicum"*
(USP, 4th rev., p. 22).
Catechu
"An extract prepared principally from the wood of Acacia
Catechu"* (USP, 4th rev., p. 23).
Cera Alba
"Yellow wax, bleached" (USP, 4th rev., p. 23).
Ceratum Adipis
Lard
White wax
Ceratum Resinae
Resin
Yellow wax
Lard
Chlorinium (materials for preparing in a package)
Black oxide of manganese*
Muriatic acid
Distilled water
Chloroformum Purificatum
Commercial chloroform
Sulfuric acid
Stronger alcohol
Potassium carbonate
Chloroformum venale
Chlorinated lime
Slaked lime
Sulfuric acid
Calcium chloride
Distilled water
Cinchona Calisayae Pulvis
"The bark of Cinchona Calisaya, called in commerce *Calisaya bark,*
and not containing less than two per cent of alkaloids yielding
crystallizable salts"* (USP, 4th rev., p. 25).

Cinchoniae Sulphas
 Mother-water remaining after quinine sulfate crystallized
 Solution of soda
 Alcohol
 Dilute sulfuric acid
 Animal charcoal*
Collodium
 Cotton
 Potassium nitrate*
 Sulfuric acid
 Stronger ether
 Stronger alcohol
Copaiba
 "The juice of Copaifera multijuga and of other species of Copaifera"
 (USP, 4th rev., p. 26).
Creasotum
 "A peculiar substance obtained from wood-tar."* (USP, 4th rev.,
 p. 26). (Much of the creosote used in pharmacy during the Civil War
 did not meet the officinal description; it was German-made from
 coal tar, not from wood.)
Creta Preparata
 Chalk*
 Water
Cubebae Oleo-resina
 Cubeb* in fine powder
 Ether
Cupri Sulphas (Blue vitriol)
 Copper sulfate in blue crystals
Extractum Aconiti Radicis Fluidum (Among the medicines dismissed
 from USP, 4th rev. See, p. 371.)
 Aconite root*
 Alcohol
Extractum Belladonnae
 Belladonna leaf* in fine powder
 Alcohol
 Diluted alcohol

Extractum Buchu Fluidum
  Buchu (dried leaves)* in moderately fine powder
  Alcohol
Extractum Cinchonae Fluidum (with aromatics)
  Yellow cinchona*
  Sugar
  Diluted alcohol
  Cinnamon*
  Ginger*
  Cardamom*
  Nutmeg*
Extractum Colchici Seminis Fluidum
  Colchicum seed*
  Alcohol
Extractum Colocynthidis Compositum
  Fluid extract of colocynth
    Colocynthis*
      "The fruit, deprived of its rind, of Citrullus Colocynthis"*
      (USP, 4th rev., p. 26).
  Socotrine aloes*
  Resin of scammony*
  Cardamom*
  Soap in fine powder
Extractum Conii
  Hemlock leaves
  Water
Extractum Ergotae Fluidum
  Ergot*
  Acetic acid
  Diluted alcohol
Extractum Gentianae Fluidum
  The root of *Gentiana lutea**
  Diluted alcohol
Extractum Glycyrrhizae
  Root of *Glycyrrhiza glabra**
  Alcohol

Extractum Hyoscyami
  Henbane leaf
  Water
Extractum Ipecacuanhae Fluidum
  The root of *Cephaelis Ipecacuanhae**
  Acetic acid
  Alcohol
Extractum Nucis Vomicae
  Seed of *Strychnos Nux vomica**
  Alcohol
Extractum Pruni Virginianae Fluidum
  Wild-cherry bark
  Sweet almond*
  Sugar
  Alcohol
Extractum Rhei Fluidum
  "The root of Rheum palmatum, and of other species of
  Rheum"* (USP, 4th rev., p. 46).
  Sugar
  Alcohol
Extractum Senegae Fluidum
  Root of *Polygala senega* (Seneka)
  Diluted alcohol
Extractum Spigeliae Fluidum
  Root of *Spigelia marilandica* (Pinkroot)
  Sugar
  Diluted alcohol
Extractum Valerianae Fluidum
  Root of *Valeriana officinalis** in fine powder
  Alcohol
Extractum Veratri Viridis Fluidum
  Root of American hellebore in fine powder
  Alcohol
Extractum Zingiberis Fluidum
  Rhizome of ginger* in fine powder
  Alcohol

Ferri Chloridi Tinctura
    Iron wire
    Muratic acid
    Nitric acid
Ferri Iodidi Syrupus
    Iodine*
    Iron wire
    Distilled water
    Syrup
Ferri Oxidum Hydratum
    Liquor ferri per sulphatis
    Ammonia water
    Water
Ferri Persulphatis Liquor (Monsel's solution)
    Iron sulfate
    Sulfuric acid
    Nitric acid
    Distilled water
Ferri Persulphatis Pulvis
    Liquor ferri per sulphatis
    Ammonia water
Ferri et Quiniae Citras
    Iron citrate in solution
    Citric acid
    Ammonia water
    Distilled water
    Tersulfate of iron
        Tersulfate of iron
            Sulfuric acid
            Nitric acid
            Water
            Iron sulfate
                Iron sulfate (Green vitriol)
                    Iron wire
                    Diluted sulfuric acid
    Quinine sulfate
    Diluted sulfuric acid

Ammonia water
Distilled water
Ferri Sulphas (Green vitriol)
   See above, Ferri et quiniae citras
Glycerina
   Soap makers' waste or lard
   Water
   Lime
Glycyrrhizae Pulvis
   Powdered root of *Glycyrrhiza glabra**
Hydrargyri Chloridum Corrosivum (Corrosive sublimate)
   Mercury
   Sulfuric acid
   Sodium chloride
   Distilled water
Hydrargyri Chloridum Mite[†]
   Mercury
   Sulfuric acid
   Sodium chloride
   Distilled water
Hydrargyri Iodidum Flavum (not in USP, 4th rev.).
   "Protonitrate or some other protosalt of mercury"
   Potassium iodide*
   Iodine*
Hydrargyri Oxidum Rubrum (Red Precipitate)
   Mercury
   Nitric acid
   Water
Hydrargyri Pilulae (Blue pills)
   Mercury
   Licorice root*
   Confection of rose*
      Confection of rose
         Red rose in fine powder (*Rose gallica**)
         Sugar
         Clarified honey

[†]This was omitted from the May 7, 1863, edition of the supply table.

Rose water
     Rose water
          Pale rose (*Rose centifolia**)
          Water
Hydrargyri Unguentum
     Mercury
     Lard
     Suet
Hydrargyri Unguentum Nitratis
     Mercury
     Nitric acid
     Neat's-foot oil
     Lard
Hydrargyrum Cum Creta
     Mercury
     Prepared chalk*
Iodinium*
     Kelp*
     Sulfuric oxide
     Manganese oxide
Ipecacuanhae et Opii Pulvis (Dover's powder)
     Ipecacuanhae* in fine powder
     Opium* dried and in fine powder
     Potassium sulfate
          Potassium sulfate
               Saltpeter*
               Sulfuric acid
Ipecacuanhae Pulvis*
     See above, Extractum ipecacuanhae
Lini Pulvis
     Powdered linseed; seeds ground but not deprived of their oil
     by expression
Linum
     Flaxseed (USP, 4th rev., p. 34).
Magnesia (Magnesium carbonate)
     Carbonate of soda
     Magnesium sulfate or bittern of salt works
     Distilled water

Magnesium Sulphas (Epsom salt)
   Magnesite or dolomite
   Sulfuric acid
Morphia Sulphas
   Distilled water
   Diluted sulfuric acid
   Morphia
      Morphia
         Opium*
         Ammonia water
         Animal charcoal
         Alcohol
         Distilled water
Olei Menthae Piperitae Tincture
   Fresh peppermint
   Water
Oleum Cinnamomi*
   Cinnamon bark*
   Water
Oleum Morrhuae
   "The fixed oil obtained from the liver of Gadus Morrhua, and other species of Gadus" (USP, 4th rev., p. 39).
Oleum Olivae
   "The oil obtained from the fruit of Olea Europea"* (USP, 4th rev., p. 40).
Oleum Ricini
   "The oil obtained from the seed of Ricinus communis"* (USP, 4th rev., p. 40).
Oleum Terebinthinae
   "The volatile oil distilled from the turpentine of Pinus palustris and of other species of Pinus"* (USP, 4th rev., p. 40).
Oleum Tiglii
   "The oil obtained from the seed of *Croton Tiglium*"* (USP, 4th rev., p. 41).
Opii Pulvis
   Powdered opium*

Opii Tinctura
  Opium*
  Alcohol
  Diluted alcohol
  Water
Opii Tinctura Camphorata
  Opium*
  Camphor*
  Oil of anise*
  Clarified honey
  Diluted alcohol
  Benzoic acid
    Benzoic acid
      Benzoin*
Pilulae Camphorae et Opii
  Camphor*
  Opium,* powdered
  Alcohol
  Confection of rose*
Pilulae Catharticae Compositae
  Compound extract of colocynth
  Mild chloride of mercury
  Gamboge*
  Extract of Jalap
    Extract of Jalap
      Jalap*
      Alcohol
      Water
Pilulae Opii
  Opium*
  Soap
Plumbi Acetas (Sugar of lead)
  Acetic acid
  Litharge (lead oxide)
Podophylli Resina
  Mayapple rhizome in fine powder
  Alcohol
  Water

Potassae Acetas
    Acetic acid
    Potassium bicarbonate (saleratus)
Potassae Bicarbonas
    Distilled water
    Potassium carbonate
    Carbonic acid
      Carbonic acid
        Dilute sulfuric acid
        Marble or bicarbonate of soda
          Sodium bicarbonate*
            Sodium carbonate
            Carbonic acid
              Sodium carbonate
                Sodium chloride
                Sulfuric acid
                Chalk*
                Animal charcoal or from kelp* or barilla*
Potassae Bitartras (Cream of Tartar)
    Potassium carbonate
    Hydrated lime
    Chlorine
Potassae Chloras
    Potassium carbonate
    Hydrated lime
    Chlorine
Potassae Nitras
    Nitre or saltpeter*
Potassii Iodidum
    Potassium (potash)
    Iodine*
    Charcoal
    Distilled water
Quiniae Sulphas
    Yellow cinchona in coarse powder*
    Muriatic acid
    Lime in fine powder
    Animal charcoal*

Sulfuric acid
Alcohol
Distilled water
Rhei Pulvis
  Powdered rhubarb*
  (Rhei pulvis is not in USP, 4th rev., but Pulvis Rhei Compositus
  is listed—powdered rhubarb,* magnesia,* ginger.*)
Rheum*
  "The root of *Rheum palmatum,* and of other species of *Rheum*"*
  (USP, 4th rev., p. 46).
Sapo
  Soda (pearlash)
  Olive oil
Scillae Pulvis
  Squill,* powdered
Scillae Syrupus
  Sugar
  Vinegar of squill
    Vinegar of squill
      Powdered squill*
      Diluted acetic acid
Sinapis Nigris Pulvis
  "The seed of Sinapis nigra"* (USP, 4th rev., p. 50).
Sodae Bicarbonas
  see above, Potassae bicarbonas
Sodae Boras
  Native borax (tincal)*
Sodae Chlorinata Liquor
  Sodium carbonate*
  Water
  Chloride of lime
    Chloride of lime
      Hydrated lime
      Chlorine
Sodae et Potassae Tartras (Rochelle salt)
  Sodium carbonate*
  Cream of tartar*
  Water

Spiritus Frumenti (whiskey)
"Spirit obtained from fermented grain by distillation, and containing from forty-eight to fifty-six per cent of absolute alcohol. Whiskey for medicinal use should be free from disagreeable odor, and not less than two years old" (USP, 4th rev., p. 52).

Spiritus Lavandulae Compositus
Cinnamon*
Cloves*
Nutmeg*
Red Saunders*
"The wood of Ptericarpus santalinus"* (USP, 4th rev., p. 48).
Oil of Rosemary*
Fresh flowering tops of *Rosmarinus officinalis**
Oil of Lavender*
Flowers of *Lavandula officinalis**

Spiritus Vini Gallici (brandy)*
"Brandy for medicinal use should be not less than four years old"* (USP, 4th rev., p. 52).

Strychnia
*Nux vomica**
Lime
Muriatic acid
Alcohol
Diluted alcohol
Diluted sulfuric acid
Ammonia water
Charcoal

Sulphur (Precipitated Sulfur)
Sublimed sulfur*
Lime
Muriatic acid
Water

Vinum Album (sherry wine)*
Vinum Xericum (USP, 4th rev., p. 55).

Zinci Acetas
Zinc
Lead acetate
Distilled water

Zinci Carbonas
    Sodium carbonate*
    Water
    Zinc Sulfate
        Zinc Sulfate
           Zinc
           Sulfuric acid
           Distilled water
Zinci Chloridi Liquor
    Zinc
    Nitric acid
    Muriatic acid
    Prepared chalk*
Zinci Sulphas
    See Zinci Carbonas

Appendix B

Contents of Autenrieth Medicine Wagon

MEDICINES

$^1/_2$ lb.	Acaciae Pulvis	1 bottle
$^1/_2$ lb.	Acid Sulphur Aromat	1 bottle
1 oz.	Acid Tannicum	1 bottle
2 lbs.	Aether Fortior	4 bottles
2 qts.	Alcohol Fortius	2 bottles
6 qts.	Alcohol Fortius	1 tin can
8 oz.	Alumen	1 bottle
8 oz.	Ammoniae Carbonas	1 bottle
1 oz.	Antim. et Potassae Tartratis Pulvis	1 bottle
32 oz.	Aqua Ammoniae	2 bottles
1 oz.	Argenti Nitras	1 bottle
1 oz.	Argenti Nitras Fusus	1 bottle
4 oz.	Bismuthi Subcarbonas	1 bottle
1 oz.	Brominium	1 bottle
8 oz.	Camphora	1 bottle
4 oz.	Cera Alba	1 tin can
3 lbs.	Ceratum Adipis	3 tin cans
$^1/_2$ lb.	Ceratum Cantharidis	1 tin can
1 lb.	Ceratum Resinae	1 tin can
32 oz.	Chloroformum Purificatum	4 bottles
24 oz.	Cinchoniae Sulphas	2 bottles and 5 cans
4 oz.	Collodium	1 bottle
2 lbs.	Copaiba	2 bottles
4 oz.	Creasotum	1 bottle
2 oz.	Cupri Sulphas	1 bottle

Note: As filled at United States Army Laboratory, Philadelphia. Printed inventory in Surgeon General's Office, Letters Received.

4	oz.	Extr. Aconiti Rad. Fluidum	1 bottle
1	oz.	Extra. Belladonnae	1 bottle
16	oz.	Extra. Cinchonae Fluidum	2 bottles
4	oz.	Extra. Colchici Sem. Fluidum	1 bottle
8	oz.	Extra. Colocynth Cp. Pulv.	1 bottle
8	oz.	Extr. Ipecacuanhae Fluidum	1 bottle
8	oz.	Extr. Zingiberis Fluidum	1 bottle
2	oz.	Ferri et Quiniae Citras	1 bottle
2	oz.	Ferri Persulphatis Pulvis	1 bottle
8	oz.	Glycerina	1 bottle
8	oz.	Hydrargyri Chloridum Mite	1 bottle
8	oz.	Ipecac, et Opii Pulvis	1 bottle
12	lbs.	Lini Pulvis	1 tin can
4	fl. oz.	Liq. Ferri Subsulphatis	1 bottle
32	fl. oz.	Liquor Potassae Permanganatis	2 bottles
32	fl. oz.	Liquor Sodae Chlorinatae	2 bottles
1	lb.	Liquor Zinci Chloridi	1 bottle
14	lbs.	Magnesium Sulphas	1 tin can
$1/2$	lb.	Mass. Pilul. Hydr.	1 jar
$1/4$	oz.	Morphia Sulphas	2 bottles
2	qts.	Oleum Olivae	2 bottles
4	qts.	Oleum Ricini	4 bottles
1	qt.	Oleum Terebinthinae	1 bottle
1	oz.	Oleum Tiglii	1 bottle
8	oz.	Opii Pulvis	1 bottle
12	doz.	Pilulae Camphorae et Opii	4 bottles
16	doz.	Pilulae Catharticae Compositae	1 bottle
16	doz.	Pilulae Extr. Colocynth. et Ipecac	1 bottle
10	doz.	Pilulae Opii	1 bottle
12	doz.	Pilulae Quiniae Sulphatis	1 bottle
8	oz.	Plumbi Acetas	1 bottle
8	oz.	Potassae Bicarbonas	1 bottle
8	oz.	Potassae Chloras	1 bottle
8	oz.	Potassii Iodidum	1 bottle
12	oz.	Quiniae Sulphas	2 bottles
			2 cans
8	lbs.	Sapo	in paper
9	lbs.	Sinapis Nigris Pulvis	1 tin can
8	oz.	Sodae Bicarbonas	1 bottle
16	oz.	Sodae et Potassae Tartr.	2 bottles
16	oz.	Spiritus Aetheris Comp.	2 bottles
32	oz.	Spiritus Aetheris Nitrosi	3 bottles
4	oz.	Spiritus Ammon. Aromat	1 bottle
24	qts.	Spiritus Frumenti	24 bottles

6	qts.	Spiritus Vini Gallici	6 bottles
4	lbs.	Syrupus Scillae	4 bottles
8	oz.	Tinctura Ferri Chloridi	1 bottle
16	oz.	Tinctura Opii	2 bottles
16	oz.	Tinctura Opii Camphor	1 bottle
1	lb.	Ung. Hydrarg	1 jar
4	oz.	Ung. Hydrarg Nitratis	1 jar
1	oz.	Zinci Sulphas	1 bottle

HOSPITAL STORES

10	lbs.	Arrowroot	1 tin can
5	lbs.	Black Tea	1 tin can
2	lbs.	Candles, Sperm	in paper
15	lbs.	Crushed Sugar	1 tin can
16	lbs.	Extract of Beef	8 tin cans
12	qts.	Extract of Coffee	12 tin cans
10	lbs.	Farina	1 tin can
4	oz.	Nutmegs	1 tin can

INSTRUMENTS

1		Buck's Sponge-holder
12		Cupping Tins
2		Lancets, Thumb
1		Pocket Case
12		Probangs
2		Scarificators
2		Scissors
1		Stethoscope
1		Syringe (rubber)
6		Syringe, Penis (glass)
1		Syringe, Self-injecting
1	case	Teeth Extracting Instruments
1		Tongue Depressor (hinged)
8		Tourniquets, Field
2		Tourniquets, Screw
4		Trusses

DRESSINGS, &c.

5	yds.	Adhesive Plaster
8	pieces	Binder's Board ($2\frac{1}{2}'' \times 12''$)
8	pieces	Binder's Board ($4'' \times 17''$)
2		Cotton Bats
1	sheet	Cotton Wadding
4	yds.	Flannel, Red
2	yds.	Gutta-percha Cloth
5	yds.	Ichthyocolla Plaster
4	lbs.	Lint, Patent
2	lbs.	Lint, Scraped
10	yds.	Muslin
1	case	Needles, 25; Cotton, 1 spool; Thimbles, 1
$2\frac{1}{4}$	yds.	Oiled Muslin
$2\frac{1}{4}$	yds.	Oiled Silk
12		Pencils, Hair
2	papers	Pins
32	doz.	Roller Bandages, assorted
1	yd.	Silk, Green (for shades)
1	oz.	Silk, Surgeon's
1	set	Splints
8	oz.	Sponge, Fine
8		Suspensory Bandages
4	pieces	Tape
10	lbs.	Tow
1	doz.	Towels
8	oz.	Twine

BEDDING, &c.

20	Blankets in 2 cases
8	Gutta-percha Bed Covers

BOOKS, &c.

1		Blank Book
2		Blank Book quarto
1		Case Book
100		Envelopes
1	copy	Gun-shot Wounds—Longmore

2	bottles	Ink (2 oz. each)
1		Inkstand, Portable
1	bottle	Mucilage
1		Order and Letter Book
2	quires	Paper, Wrapping, White and Blue
4	quires	Paper, Writing
6		Pencils, Lead
12		Pens, Steel, with holders
1		Portfolio
1		Register of Patients
1	stick	Sealing Wax
1	copy	Surgery, Erichsen's
1	copy	Surgery, Smith's Handbook
1	copy	Surgery, Sargent's Minor
1	copy	U.S. Dispensatory

FURNITURE, &c.

2		Basins, Tin (small)
3		Basins, Wash, hand
1		Bed Pan, delf
2		Buckets, I. R.
10	dozen	Corks, assorted
1		Corkscrew
1		Funnel, I. R.
1		Grater, Nutmeg
1		Hatchet
1		Hone and Strop
3		Lanterns, Glass
1	box	Matches
1		Measure, graduated, 2 oz.
2		Measure, graduated, minim
2		Medicinal Measuring Glasses
1		Mill, coffee
1		Mortar and Pestle, Wedgewood
2	papers	Pill Boxes
1		Pill Tile
1		Razor and Strop (in case)
1	set	Scales and Weights, prescription
1	set	Scales and Weights, shop
1		Sheepskin, dressed
2		Spatulas, 3 and 6 in.
6		Tin Scoops
2	dozen	Urinals, delf
2		Vials, assorted

Appendix C

Contents of U.S. Army
Medicine Pannier (Squibb)

*The following is verbatim text of a broadside that arrived in the field
with each pannier packed by E. R. Squibb. The original broadside
shows a diagram listing each drug title Nos. 1 to 52, within a separate
square corresponding exactly, in its relative position, to the compart-
ment for the drug in the pannier itself. This standardized layout of the
packed drugs, together with the diagram, assured quick selection of a
needed drug and minimized risk of error.*

The Pannier should always be kept top up and handled with care. It
should be carefully protected from the sun and rain because either heat
or moisture will cause many of the pills to flatten and run together,
whilst if the pills be dried so hard as to protect them against such
contingencies they are liable to pass through the alimentary canal without dissolving and therefore without effect.

When not in frequent use or when to be transported to a distance the
screws of the iron plate in front should be put in; but when to be used
frequently they should be taken out and kept inside. The Pannier should
always be kept locked when not in use and the key in the possession of
the medical officer or hospital steward.

When the Pannier is to be carried on the back of a horse or mule, it
may be attached to the Packsaddle by ropes either on the top of the
Saddle or on one side if counterbalanced by a pack of equal weight. It
should however always be carried high on the Saddle so as not to press
the side of the animal.

As the labels of the bottles cannot be seen while the bottles are in
their places the following diagram will facilitate the finding of any

particular bottle and with the list below it will serve as an inventory of the original contents of the Pannier.

The bottles should always be kept in the places indicated in the diagram and when taken out by the aid of the diagram should be carefully identified by the label or by the number, if the label be lost or defaced, to prevent mistakes from bottles getting misplaced.

Where the simple officinal latin name is used upon the label the strictly officinal preparation is indicated. But when any departure from the official standard is required, the variation is explained upon the label, as in the instance of Pilula Quiniae Sulphatis, which name would indicate the officinal pills of one grain each, except that the explanatory line upon the label states that these contain three grains each. Where english names are used, the indication is that the preparation is not officinal, and in these cases the formula is unvariably placed upon the label.

The Whiskey when kept in tinned iron vessels for some time is liable to be blackened by a chemical reaction between the acids of the whiskey and the iron. This discoloration is not hurtful.

The Liquor Ferri Persulphatis and Collodium should be kept carefully stopped with corks, because glass stoppers soon become so fixed as to render the contents of the bottles inaccessible.

The tow in which the bottles and other articles are packed is not necessarily to be replaced, for ordinary Army or field transportation, provided proper care be taken of the Pannier, that as much of the tow as possible should be kept in the Pannier in case of need for surgical uses.

1. CERATUM CANTHARIDIS. Three ounces
2. ARGENTI NITRAS. One ounce
3. ARGENTI NITRAS FUSUS. One ounce
4. IODINIUM. One ounce
5. ANTIMONII ET POTASSAE TARTRAS. One ounce
6. HYDRARGYRI CHLORIDUM MITE. One ounce
7. EXTRACT OF BEEF. One pound
8. EXTRACT OF COFFEE. One pound
9. CONDENSED MILK. One pound
10. BLACK TEA. Four ounces
11. SPIRITUS FRUMENTI. Twenty four fluidounces
12. SPIRITUS AETHERIS NITRICI. Eight fluidounces

13. ALCOHOL FORTIUS. Twelve fluidounces
14. COUGH MIXTURE. Twelve fluidounces
15. WHITE SUGAR. Ten ounces
16. CHLOROFORMUM PURIFICATUM. Twelve fluidounces
17. LINIMENT. Twelve fluidounces
18. SYRUPUS SCILLAE. Eight fluidounces
19. AQUA AMMONIAE. Eight fluidounces
20. SPIRITUS AETHERIS COMPOSITUS. Four fluidounces
21. TINCTURA OPII. Six fluidounces
22. EXTRACTUM CINCHONAE FLUIDUM. with Aromatics   Four fluidounces
23. EXTRACTUM VALERIANAE FLUIDUM. Six fluidounces
24. EXTRACTUM ZINGIBERIS FLUIDUM. Six fluidounces
25. OLEUM OLIVAE. Six fluidounces
26. OLEUM TEREBINTHINAE. Six fluidounces
27. GLYCERINA. Six fluidounces
28. TINCTURA OPII CAMPHORATA. Six fluidounces
29. LIQUOR FERRI PERSULPHATUS. Four fluidounces
30. SPIRITUS AMMONIAE AROMATICUS. Four fluidounces
31. PILULAE CATHARTICAE COMPOSITAE. Fifty dozen
32. PILLS OF COLOCYNTII AND IPECAC. Fifty dozen
33. PULVIS IPECAC: ET OPII. in five gram pills   Thirty dozen
34. PILULAE QUINIAE: SULPHATIS. three grams each   Forty dozen
35. POTASSAE CHLORAS. Four ounces
36. POTASSAE BICARBONAS. Four ounces
37. POTASSII IODIDUM. Four ounces
38. SODAE ET POTASSAE TARTRAS. Four ounces
39. LIQUOR MORPHIAE SULPHATIS. sixteen grains to the fluidounce. Four fluidounces
40. PILLS OF CAMPHOR AND OPIUM. Twenty dozen
41. PILULAE HYDRARGYRI. Forty dozen
42. PILULAE OPII. Sixty dozen
43. ACIDUM TANNICUM. Half an ounce
44. ALUMEN. Three ounces
45. COLLODIUM. Three fluidounces
46. CREASOTUM. Two fluidounces
47. EXTRACTUM ACONITI RADICIS FLUIDUM. Three fluidounces
48. EXTRACTUM COLCHICI SEMINIS FLUIDUM. Three fluidounces
49. EXTRACTUM IPECACUANHAE FLUIDUM. Three fluidounces
50. TINCTURA FERRI CHLORIDI. Two fluidounces

51. PLUMBI ACETAS. Three ounces
52. ZINCI SULPHAS. Three ounces

Besides the articles enumerated above the trays contain the following:

CERATUM ADIPIS one pound
SAPO one cake
UNGUENTUM HYDRARGYRI six
   ounces

INSTRUMENTS

CUPPING TINS four
PROBANG one
SCISSORS one
SYRINGES, self injecting—one
SYRINGES PENIS, glass—four
TOURNIQUETS, Field—two

DRESSINGS, &c.

ADHESIVE PLASTER two yards
BINDERS BOARD eight pieces
ICHTHYOCOLLA PLASTER one
   yard
LINT, Patent half a pound
MATCHES one box
MUSLIN three yards
NEEDLES 25 COTTON 1 spool
THIMBLE, 1, in one case
OILED SILK seven eighth of a yard
PENCILS hair, in a vial, six
PINS one paper
ROLLER BANDAGES, assorted
   three doz.
SADDLERS SILK a quarter oz.
SPONGE, dressing six pieces

TAPE two inches
TOW one pound

BOOKS, &c.

BLANK BOOKS, small two
NOTE PAPER two quires
ENVELOPES twenty five
INKSTAND, travellers, one
PENS Steel twelve
PENHOLDERS three
PENCILS, lead two
TIN TRAY for STATIONERY one

FURNITURE, &c.

BASINS, dressing two
CANDLES half pound
CANDLE HOLDER one
CORKS four doz.
CORKSCREW one
MEASURE, graduated one
MEASURE, minim one
MEDICINE MEASURING GLASS
   one
MORTAR and PESTLE one
PILL BOXES half a paper
SCALES and WEIGHTS one set
SPATULA one
TEASPOON one
TOWELS three
VIALS six

Notes

The following abbreviations are used.

AGO	Adjutant General's Office
AJP	*American Journal of Pharmacy*
Druggists' Circular	*American Druggists' Circular and Chemical Gazette*
Hammond court martial trial	Hammond court martial trial, Records of the Judge Advocate General, MM 1430, Record Group 153, National Archives
MSH	*The Medical and Surgical History of the War of the Rebellion*
OR	*The War of the Rebellion: A Compilation of the Official Records of the Union and Confederate Armies*
SG Letterbooks	Surgeon General's Letterbooks
SGO	Surgeon General's Office
USD	*The Dispensatory of the United States of America*
USP	*The Pharmacopoeia of the United States of America*

Preface

1. Glenn Sonnedecker, "Foreword," in George Winston Smith, *Medicines for the Union Army* (Madison, WI: American Institute of the History of Pharmacy, 1962), p. v.

Chapter 1

1. "Editorial Department," *American Journal of Pharmacy,* Vol. 37 (January 1865), p. 75.
2. Frederick De Block, "Military Medicine in the Eighteenth Century," *The Military Surgeon,* Vol. 65 (October 1919), pp. 561-565.

3. Fielding H. Garrison, *An Introduction to the History of Medicine* (Philadelphia, W. B. Saunders & Co., 1914), pp. 327-328.

4. Louis C. Duncan, *The Medical Department in the Civil War* (binder's title [n.p., no pub., n.d.]), "The Comparative Mortality of Disease and Battle Casualties in the Historical Wars of the World," pp. 22-23. This volume is not paged consecutively throughout but separately by chapters; page references will be to the paging within the chapters.

5. Ibid., p. 25.

6. The bed capacity of these 192 hospitals was 118,057 on December 17, 1864. See Charles Smart, "The General Hospitals," in *The Medical* and *Surgical History of the War of the Rebellion,* 6 Volumes, (Washington, D.C., Government Printing Office, 1870-1888), Part III, Vol. 2, p. 964. Brevet Major General Joseph K. Barnes, Surgeon General of the United States Army, "Report of the Surgeon General [1865]," *House Executive Documents,* Vol. 3, 39th Congress, 1st Session, p. 896.

7. These statistics understate the total number of sick and wounded. They do not include prisoners of war, those absent from their commands, those present and accounted for who did not file sick reports, or the "floating population" of the hospitals. See MSH, Part III, Vol. 1, pp. 3-4.

8. Ibid., pp. 79, 191, 624, 751, 891. During the period that figures were collected for Negro troops, there were among the 186,000 Negro soldiers: 159,670 cases of malaria, 11,746 cases of typhoid fever, and 8,555 cases of measles. The venereal disease rate was lower among the Negro soldiers than among the white troops.

9. M. A. Reasoner, "The Development of the Medical Supply Service," *The Military Surgeon,* Vol. 63 (July 1928), p. 5.

10. Duncan, *Medical Department,* "The Comparative Mortality of Disease and Battle Casualties," p. 37; see also, "Medical Department of the Army During the War," *American Druggists' Circular and Chemical Gazette,* Vol. 9 (July 1865), p. 151.

11. George Worthington Adams, *Doctors in Blue: The Medical History of the Union Army in the Civil War* (New York, H. Schuman, 1952), p. 228.

12. "Army Hospital Supplies," *The American Medical Times,* cited in *Druggists' Circular,* Vol. 7 (April 1863), p. 76.

13. For a complete list, together with the constituent elements of the pharmaceutical preparations, see Appendix A.

14. "Abstract 'A,' Statement of the quantity of medical supplies issued during the war from the purveying depots at New York City, Philadelphia, Penn., Baltimore, Md., Washington, D.C., Cincinnati, Ohio, Louisville, Ky., and St. Louis, Mo.," Report of the Secretary of War, 1866, *House Executive Documents,* Vol. 3, 39th Congress, 2nd Session, p. 384. Medical supplies were sent from the central purveying depots in Philadelphia and New York City to the other depots before being forwarded either to the armies in the field or to the general hospitals. It is possible, therefore, that these figures may in some instances be too great because the medicines may have been counted in more than one depot. The figures given

differ somewhat but not excessively from those presented in a tabular statement of "Supplies purchased and manufactured during the war by the Medical Department of the Army," by surgeon W. C. Spencer in MSH. Spencer's list is not as complete as the one used here. See MSH, Part III, Vol. 1, p. 966.

15. "Statement of the Quantity of Medical Supplies," p. 385.

16. Adams, *Doctors in Blue,* p. 227.

17. George B. Wood and Franklin Bache, *The Dispensatory of the United States of America* (Eleventh Edition, Philadelphia, J. B. Lippincott Co., 1858), p. 439.

18. "Statement of the Quantity of Medical Supplies," p. 384

19. Ibid.; *The Pharmacopoeia of the United States of America* (Fourth Decennial Revision, Philadelphia, J. B. Lippincott & Co., 1863), pp. 368-369.

20. "Statement of the Quantity of Medical Supplies," p. 384.

21. Congressional appropriations are in some respects an inaccurate gauge of the financial limitations of the Medical Department since during 1861 more money was spent on medical supplies than was appropriated. Nevertheless, for the fiscal year ending June 30, 1861, Congress appropriated $76,225.50. For the expenses of that department for the year ending June 30, 1862 "to meet circumstances growing out of the rebellion of the Southern States," the appropriation was $115,000. During the fiscal year ending June 30, 1861, $174,037.88 was actually expended for medical and hospital supplies. As a comparison, $10,566,321.03 was spent in the fiscal year ending June 30, 1863 on account of medicines, instruments, hospital stores, bedding, and other supplies. *The War of the Rebellion: A Compilation of the Official Records of the Union and Confederate Armies,* 129 volumes and index (Washington, Government Printing Office, 1880-1901), Series III, Vol. 1, p. 634; Vol. 3, p. 964.

22. MSH, Part III, Vol. 1, p. 964.

23. See Finley's report of the activities of the surgeon general's office, November 13, 1861, in OR, Series III, Vol. 1, pp. 633-636.

24. *Revised Regulations for the Army of the United States, 1861* (Philadelphia, J. B. Lippincott & Co., 1861), pp. 292-309.

25. MSH, Part III, Vol. 1, p. 964.

26. Before the war, Hammond had been able to secure the addition of Bibron's antidote for snake bite to the army supply table. See S. Weir Mitchell, "Inquiry into the Correctness of the Belief that Prof. Bibron was the Inventor of the Antidote which bears his Name," *The American Journal of Medical Sciences,* Vol. 48 (October 1864), p. 420.

27. L. A. Edwards, By Order of the Surgeon General, to Satterlee, June 17, 1862 (fair copy), Surgeon General's Letterbooks, Military Letters, Record Group 112, National Archives.

28. *Directions Concerning the Manner of Obtaining and Accounting for Medical and Hospital Supplies for the Army with a Standard Supply Table* (Washington, Government Printing Office, 1862), pp. 7-9; MSH, Part III, Vol. 1, p. 964.

29. *Directions Concerning the Duties of Medical Purveyors and Medical Storekeepers and the Manner of Obtaining and Accounting for Medical and Hos-*

pital Supplies for the Army, with a Supply Table (Circular No. 7, Washington, Government Printing Office, 1863), p. 31. For the controversy over calomel and tartar emetic, see "Calomel and Tartar Emetic in the Army," *The American Medical Times,* Vol. 6 (June 20, 1863), pp. 297-298; "Removal of Calomel and Tartar Emetic," ibid., pp. 298-299.

30. *Revised Regulations, 1861,* p. 281.

31. Alex Berman, "A Striving for Scientific Respectability," *Bulletin of the History of Medicine,* Vol. 30 (January-February 1956), pp. 7, 18-19. One New York jobber told Guthrie in the late 1850s that he was often swamped with orders for the indigenous drugs. See C. B. Guthrie, "Some Remarks in Regard to Our Indigenous Materia Medica," *Proceedings of the American Pharmaceutical Association* Vol. 7(1858), p. 432.

32. John Uri Lloyd and C. G. Lloyd, "Cercis," *Drugs and Medicines of North America,* 2 vols. (Cincinnati, J.U. Lloyd and C.G. Lloyd, 1884-1887), Vol. 2, p. 125. (Reproduced in the Bulletin Series of the Lloyd Library of Botany, Pharmacy and Materia Medica, Reproduction Series, No. 9, Vol. 2.) There probably was no shortage at Cairo of preparations on the supply table. The general hospital there had "an apothecary's room supplied with an ample store of medicines and surgical appliances." See Mary A. Livermore, *My Story of the War* (Hartford, Connecticut, A. D. Worthington and Company, 1890), p. 204.

33. "Petroleum in Surgery," *Druggists' Circular,* Vol. 8 (June 1863), p. 155.

34. OR, Series I, Vol. 5, p. 79.

35. Ibid., pp. 79-80.

36. Ibid., p. 83.

37. Hammond to Letterman, June 19, 1862, cited in P. M. Ashburn, *A History of the Medical Department of the United States Army* (Boston, Houghton Mifflin, 1929), p. 77. Hammond's Circular of October 20, 1862, directed the surgeons as follows: "The standard of medical and hospital supplies for the Army is the following supply table. It is not the design of the Department to confine medical officers absolutely to that table, either in variety or quantity, but only to establish a standard for their guidance in making requisitions for supplies, leaving individual preferences to be indulged in at the discretion of the Medical Director or the Surgeon General. Neither is it supposed that the quantities of the table will always meet the necessities of unusual emergencies, as during epidemics or in unhealthy seasons and localities. . . ." Cited in MSH, Part III, Vol. 1, p. 965.

38. *Revised Regulations, 1861,* p. 281.

39. MSH, Part III, Vol. 1, p. 964.

40. Joseph K. Barnes, Acting Surgeon General, to E. M. Stanton, Secretary of War, October 31, 1863, Surgeon General's Report Book, Record Group 112, National Archives; MSH, Part III, Vol. 1, p. 964; Hennell Stevens, "The Medical Purveying Department of the United States Army," AJP, Vol. 37 (March 1865), pp. 92-93. Throughout 1863, medical and hospital supplies valued at $5 million passed through the depot at Washington. See "Jottings," *New York Evening Post* (semiweekly edition), April 5, 1864.

41. *A Statement of the Causes Which Led to the Dismissal of Surgeon General William A. Hammond from the Army* (New York, [no pub.], 1864), p. 63.

42. [William Procter Jr.] "Editorial Department," AJP, Vol 34 (January 1862), p. 94. This article presumably was written by the editor, Procter, but it was unsigned and may have come from the pen of John M. Maisch, who had similar ideas on the subject. See also "Report on the Progress of Pharmacy," *Proceedings of the American Pharmaceutical Association,* 1862, pp. 49-50.

43. On these attitudes and the comparative newness of the pharmaceutical profession, see "The Relations of Physicians and Druggists," *Druggists' Circular,* Vol. 8 (June 1864), p. 107; George Urdang, "One Hundred and Twenty-Five Years of the Pharmacopoeia," in Solomon R. Kagan, Ed., *Victor Robinson Memorial Volume* (New York, Froben Press, 1949), p. 400. Pharmacy was not the only profession that failed to win recognition from the Medical Department of the United States Army. *The New York Dental Journal* proposed that a dental department be created in the Medical Department with a dental surgeon general at its head, but the suggestion was not accepted. See "Dental Department of the Army," *The New York Dental Journal,* cited in *The American Medical Times,* Vol. 3 (July 20, 1861), p. 48.

44. *Statutes at Large,* 37th Congress, 2nd Session, pp. 403-404; Lorenso Thomas, Adjutant General, General Orders No. 55, May 24, 1862, Adjutant General's Office, cited in OR Series III, Vol. 2, p. 67; Henry N. Rittenhouse, "U.S. Army Medical Storekeepers," AJP, Vol. 37 (March 1865), pp. 87-90.

45. Hammond to Stanton, November 10, 1862, Surgeon General's Report Book: OR, Series III, Vol. 2, p. 752.

46. Stevens, "Medical Purveying System," p. 92.

47. Edward Kremers and George Urdang, *History of Pharmacy* (1940 edition, Philadelphia, Lippincott, 1940), p. 317.

48. Adams, *Doctors in Blue,* p. 5. Although the United States Sanitary Commission usually provided supplies for the troops it also bought a few medicines for them early in the war. See William Quentin Maxwell, *Lincoln's Fifth Wheel* (New York, Longman's, Green and Co., 1956), p. 86.

49. Ibid., p. 235; *Revised Regulations, 1861,* p. 281.

50. OR, Series I, Vol. 27, part 1, p. 26.

51. Edward B. Fell, "The Pharmaceutical Department of a U.S.A. Hospital," AJP, Vol. 37 (March 1865), pp. 107-112. For descriptions of Mower General Hospital, see OR, Series III, Vol. 5, p. 240; MSH, Part III, Vol. 1, p. 932.

52. "T. M. Sharp's Positive Cure for Dyspepsia," lithograph by Peter S. Duval & Son, 1864, Library of Congress.

53. "Holloway's Pills and Ointments," lithograph by George Schlegel, 1863, Library of Congress.

54. Order of Major General E. S. Rosecrans cited in *Nashville Union,* August 2, 1863.

55. Advertisement in *Nashville Union,* June 17, 1864.

56. Hammond to Lincoln, February 13, 1863; Meredith Clymer to Hammond, February 14, 1863, Lincoln MSS., Vol. 102, Library of Congress.

57. Duncan, *Medical Department,* "Campaign of Fredericksburg," pp. 6-7.
58. Reasoner, "Medical Supply Service," p. 18; MSH, Part III, Vol. 1, p. 964.
59. MSH, Part III, Vol. 1, pp. 917-918. The medical contents of a Perot wagon were as follows: 1 oval keg (6 gallon capacity) of whiskey; stronger ether for anesthesia, 32 oz.; sweet spirit of niter, 32 oz.; solution of ammonia, 32 oz.; turpentine, 1 qt.; castor oil, 4 qts.; brandy, 6 qts.; olive oil, 2 qts.; purified chloroform, 32 oz.; copaiba, 32 oz.; quinine sulfate, 10 oz.; Syrup of Squill, 4 lbs.; aromatic sulfuric acid, tannic acid, spirit of nitrous ether, strong alcohol, alum, aromatic spirit of ammonia, Dover's powder, sulfate of morphia, laudanum, paregoric, acetate of lead, potassium bicarbonate, creasote, fluid extract of colchicum seed, fluid extract of aconite root, fluid extract of ipecac, fluid extract of senega, tincture of chloride of iron, solution of subsulfate of iron, pure glycerin, potassium chlorate, potassium iodide, bicarbonate of soda, whiskey, blue mass, citrine ointment, powdered squill, Hoffmann's anodyne, carbonate of ammonia, camphor, collodion, copper sulfate, alcoholic extract of belladonna, fluid extract of cinchona (aromatic), fluid extract of ginger, mercury and chalk, croton oil, potassium permanganate, Fowler's solution, chlorinated solution of soda, zinc chloride solution, resin cerate, simple cerate, powdered gum arabic, silver nitrate (crystals), fused silver nitrate, cinchona sulfate, citrate of iron and quinine, powdered subsulfate of iron, iodide of iron, powdered ipecac, powdered opium, camphor (2 grains) and opium (1 grain) pills, compound cathartic pills, quinine sulfate pills, quinine sulfate, powdered Rochelle salt, zinc sulfate, blistering cerate, powdered compound extract of colocynth, fluid extract of ipecac.
60. For the contents of these wagons as described by John M. Maisch, see Appendix B.
61. W. C. Spencer, By Order of the Surgeon General, to Colonel Charles McDougall, October 23, 1865 (fair copy), SG Letterbooks, Military Letters.
62. Id. to Satterlee, August 29, 1865 (fair copy), SG Letterbooks, Military Letters.
63. MSH. Part III, Vol. 1, p. 915; Hammond to Cooper, August 11, 1862, in Hammond court martial trial. On the older medicine chests, see Serry Wood, *The Old Apothecary Shop* (Watkins Glen, New York, Century House, 1956), p. 5.
64. Squibb to Satterlee, November 7, 13, 1862, Surgeon General's Office, Letters Received, Record Group 112, National Archives. See also Appendix C.
65. Reasoner, "Medical Supply Service," p. 18. When Sherman marched from Atlanta to Savannah in 1864, he took with him one medicine wagon for each division, and a pack mule loaded with medical supplies for every regiment. See Duncan, *Medical Department,* "When Sherman Marched Down to the Sea," p. 22.
66. MSH, Part III, Vol. 1, p. 915.
67. Squibb made subcontracts with Gail Borden to supply these items. See Squibb to Satterlee, November 13, 1862, SGO, Letters Received. On Borden and his products, see "Note—Borden's Extract of Beef," AJP, Vol. 38 (January 1866), pp. 81-82; "Condensed Coffee," *The American Agriculturist,* Vol. 20 (September 1861), p. 259; Joe B. Frantz, *Gail Borden, Dairyman to a Nation* (Norman, University of Oklahoma Press, 1951), pp. 258-262.

68. Squibb to Satterlee, November 13, 1862, SGO; see also Appendix C.

69. Squibb to Hammond, March 24, April 6, 1863, SGO, Letters Received.

70. MSH, Part III, Vol. 1, p. 914; *Revised Regulations, 1861*, p. 291.

71. "Correspondence: Reorganization of the Medical Staff," *The Army and Navy Journal*, Vol. 2 (August 5, 1865), p. 790.

72. It was published by Lippincott in 1862. *Proceedings of the American Pharmaceutical Association*, 1862, p. 61.

73. *Revised Regulations, 1861*, pp. 282-284.

74. Duncan, *Medical Department*, "The Battle of Bull Run," p. 22.

75. OR, Series III, Vol. 2, p. 22.

76. *The American Annual Cyclopaedia, 1862* (New York, D. Appleton & Company, 1863), pp. 17-18.

77. Duncan, *Medical Department*, "Evolution of the Ambulance Corps and Field Hospital," pp. 27-28.

78. *Revised Regulations, 1861*, p. 288n.

79. Charles Beneulyn Johnson, *Muskets and Medicine, or Army Life in the Sixties* (Philadelphia, F. A. Davis Company, 1917), pp. 127-128.

80. M. I. Wilbert, "Scientific Meeting at the Philadelphia College of Pharmacy," AJP, Vol. 75 (November 1903), p. 521.

81. "Obituary, James Vernor," *Journal of the American Pharmaceutical Association*, Vol. 16 (November 1927), p. 1124.

82. "Obituary, Joseph Lyon Lemberger," *Journal of the American Pharmaceutical Association*, Vol. 16 (October 1927), pp. 1007-1008; Joseph W. England, Ed., *The First Century of the Philadelphia College of Pharmacy, 1821-1921* (Philadelphia, The Philadelphia College of Pharmacy and Science, 1922), p. 179.

83. "Obituaries, George W. Kennedy," AJP, Vol. 75 (April 1903), p. 196.

84. OR, Series I, Vol. 19, part 1, p. 114.

85. Reasoner, "Medical Supply Service," p. 18; Duncan, *Medical Department*, "Evolution of the Ambulance Corps and Field Hospital," p. 26.

86. Reasoner, "Medical Supply Service," p. 16.

87. See for example, "Consolidated Statement of Articles and Quantities of Medical and Hospital Supplies Carried with the Army of the Potomac Across the Rapidan, May 4, 1864," OR, Series I, Vol. 36, part 1, pp. 222-223.

88. OR, Series III, Vol. 2, p. 752.

89. OR, Series I, Vol. 5, p. 80.

90. Fred B. Ryons, "The U.S. Army Medical Department, 1861-1865," *The Military Surgeon*, Vol. 29 (November 1936), p. 345; Duncan, *Medical Department*, "Evolution of the Ambulance Corps and Field Hospital," p. 16.

91. OR, Series I, Vol. II, part 1, p. 219.

92. Duncan, *Medical Department*, "Greatest Battle—Gettysburg," p. 17.

93. Ibid., "The Great Battle of Chickamauga," pp. 12, 21.

94. Cited in Victor Robinson, *White Caps: The Story of Nursing* (Philadelphia, J. B. Lippincott, 1946), p. 157. For other complaints against the medical purveying system, see "Army Medical Supplies," *The American Medical Times*, cited

in *Druggists' Circular,* Vol. 7 (April 1863), p. 76; "Army Medical Intelligence," *The Boston Medical and Surgical Journal,* Vol. 65 (December 5, 1861), p. 373.

95. Edward R. Squibb, "Permanganate of Potassa," *Druggists' Circular,* Vol. 8 (October 1864), p. 183; John H. Packard, "On Hospital Gangrene and Its Efficient Treatment," *The American Journal of Medical Sciences,* Vol. 49 (January 1865), pp. 114-119.

96. Hammond to Stanton, June 22, 1863 (fair copy), SG Letterbooks, Letters to the Secretary of War.

97. "Review of the New York Markets," *Druggists' Circular,* Vol. 5 (January 1861) p. 17.

98. Robert Swinhoe, "Formosa Camphor," *Druggists' Circular,* Vol. 8 (January 1864), p. 6.

99. "Bismuth," AJP, Vol. 38 (January 1866), pp. 87-88.

100. "Review of the New York Markets," *Druggists' Circular,* Vol. 8 (March 1864), p. 57. See also, "Drugs," Ibid. (January 1864), p. 14.

101. Ibid., "Drugs." Diplomatic relations with Great Britain were unusually critical late in 1861 during the Trent affair when the British cabinet placed a ban on the export of sulfur, saltpeter, and gunpowder to the United States. See Alfred D. Chandler Jr., "Du Pont, Dahlgren, and the Civil War Nitre Shortage," *Military Affairs,* Vol. 13 (Fall, 1949), p. 145. On monopoly control of some branches of German drug and chemical importations in Philadelphia, see "Obituary, William Henry Schively, AJP, Vol. 66 (January 1894), p. 52. At the end of 1863 most of the supply of sodium bicarbonate was held by two parties. See "Review of the New York Markets," *Druggists' Circular,* Vol. 8 (January 1864), p. 44. Camphor, the drug which next after quinine and opium was most subject to speculative variations in price, was controlled "by a few [importing] houses." Ibid., p. 14; E. Squibb, "Report on the Drug Market," *Proceedings of the American Pharmaceutical Association,* 1863, p. 179.

102. Satterlee to Surgeon General's Office, October 5, November 12, 20, December 3, 11, 31, 1863, Surgeon General's Office, Register of Letters Received, Record Group 112, National Archives.

103. "Drugs," *Druggists' Circular,* Vol. 8 (August 1864), p. 158; ibid., Vol. 9 (January 1865), p. 19.

104. Ibid. (February 1865), p. 39.

105. Squibb, "Report on the Drug Market," p. 176.

106. "Review of the New York Markets," *Druggists' Circular,* Vol. 5 (April 1861), p. 89.

107. J. Maisch, "Report on the Drug Market," *Proceedings of the American Pharmaceutical Association,* 1864, p. 189.

108. Ibid.; Squibb, "Report on the Drug Market," p. 176.

109. "Trade and Commerce," *Philadelphia North American and United States Gazette,* March 6, 1865.

110. Edward Parrish, *A Treatise on Pharmacy* (Third edition, Philadelphia, J. B. Lippincott, 1864), p. 83.

111. "Philadelphia Correspondence of the Druggists' Circular," *Druggists' Circular,* Vol. 1 (November 1857), p. 152.

112. "Review of the New York Market," *Druggists' Circular,* Vol. 8 (January 1864), p. 14; "New York Drug Exchange," ibid., p. 10.

113. "Wholesale Price Currents," *Druggists' Circular,* Vol. 8 (July 1864), p. 138. A typical transaction was described as follows: "A man pays a thousand dollars for the privilege of putting in to another a certain quantity of Gum Arabic any time within sixty days at a stipulated price. Or he pays five cents a pound down for a lot of pepper, with the privilege of taking the whole at any time within sixty days at the price agreed upon at the buyer's option. If it is not taken the money paid is lost to the buyer. . . ." Rene Leon de Milhau in his obituary of John G. Milhau declared: "During the entire war he kept close watch over the quinine market, defeating every attempt to corner the drug, so vitally necessary for the soldiers in the field." No evidence was submitted to support this statement, either by Rene Leon de Milhau or by Urdang, who apparently accepted it. See Rene Leon de Milhau, "John Milhau," *Proceedings of the American Pharmaceutical Association,* 1907, p. 581; George Urdang, *Pharmacy's Part in Society* (Madison, WI, American Institute of the History of Pharmacy, 1946), p. 22. The price of quinine, however, did remain lower than often has been claimed; the rise was much less spectacular.

114. Joseph H. Bill to Satterlee, December 31, 1864, SGO, Letters Received.

115. Joseph R. Smith, Surgeon U.S. Army, By Order of the Surgeon General, to [Stanton], January 6, 1862 (fair copy), Surgeon General's Report Books; C. H. Alden, By Order of the Surgeon General, to Satterlee, February 17, 1863 (fair copy), SG Letterbooks, Military Letters.

116. Satterlee to Hammond, March 23, 27, 28, 31, 1862 (précis, fair copies), SGO, Register of Letters Received; id. to id., March 24, 27, 1863, SGO, Letters Received; E. S. Dunster, Assistant Surgeon U.S. Army, By Order of the Surgeon General, to Robert Murray, medical purveyor, Philadelphia, July 30, 1863 (fair copy); Alden, By Order of the Surgeon General, to Satterlee, March 23, 25, 28, 1863 (fair copies); Hammond to id., March 27, 1863 (fair copy); id. to Murray, April 2, 1863 (fair copy), SG Letterbooks, Military Letters.

117. Satterlee to Hammond, March 20, 1863, SGO, Letters Received.

118. "Affidavit of John Wyeth," August 1, 1879, William A. Hammond, ACP File, Adjutant General's Office, War Department, Record Group 94, National Archives.

119. Squibb to [surgeon general's office], March 24, 1863 (précis, fair copy). SGO, Register of Letters Received.

120. R. C. Wood, Assistant Surgeon General, By Order of the Surgeon General, to Satterlee, June 7, 1862 (fair copy), SG Letterbooks, Military Letters. Even late in the war the medical purveyors were at times embarrassed by a lack of funds. See Murray to Barnes, December 3, 1864, SGO, Letters Received.

121. During the period when Hammond was Surgeon General, disbursements were made by the Medical Department in the following cities: New York City, $5,193,525.47; Philadelphia, $2,314,738.07; Louisville, $1,429,051.21; Cincin-

nati, $1,029,940.93; Baltimore, $608,320.10; St. Louis, $600,047.88. The largest amount of business was done with the following firms: Paton & Co., New York (medical supplies other than drugs), $1,813,872.90; Philip Schieffelin & Co., New York, $306,694.67; Edward R. Squibb, Brooklyn, $286,199.40; Wyeth and Brother, Philadelphia, $657,122.17; Saire, Eckstein & Co., Cincinnati, $252,122.17; Wilson & Peter, Louisville, $592,809.37. See *A Statement of the Causes Which Led to the Dismissal of Surgeon General William A. Hammond from the Army . . .* (New York, no publisher, 1864), p. 63.

122. Satterlee to J. J. B. Wright [n.d.] (fair copy in Squibb's handwriting), Squibb Notebook No. 6, May 1859-June 1861, Squibb MSS., Squibb Institute for Medical Research Library, New Brunswick, New Jersey; "Summary Statement of Supplies Purchased for the Medical and Hospital Department of the Army, from December 30, 1862 to July 20, 1863," Hammond court martial trial, Records of the Judge Advocate General, MM1430, Record Group 153, National Archives.

123. George E. Cooper testimony, February 2, 1864, Hammond court martial trial. In testifying against Hammond, Cooper said that he had told Hammond that the business of the Medical Department in Philadelphia was too much for any one supplier. He continued, "Dr. Hammond told me that when any small requisitions would come on to give them to Hance, Griffith & Co. or to T. Morris Perot & Co. and that would serve as a sop to Cerebrus and keep the people's mouths shut. He said at the same time that it was very strange that the people of Philadelphia should complain about where he made the purchases—that Dr. Satterlee of New York bought all he had to buy from Shifllein [sic] and Squibb, and nothing was said about it. That was the conversation. In consequence, I did give to [T.] Morris Perot & Co. and Hance and Griffith orders. I had purchased previously to that exclusively from Wyeth of medicines and drugs."

124. Robert Murray testimony, Hammond court martial trial. The Henry Bower firm was tied in with the Wyeth business. Bower was the only manufacturer of carbolic acid in Philadelphia, and the outstanding producer of glycerin in the East.

125. For a contemporary defense of Hammond's choice in favor of paying higher prices from manufacturers whose honesty was relied upon, see "This Week," *American Medical Times,* Vol. 7 (December 13, 1863), pp. 282-283.

126. Revelations of adulterations became so numerous and sensational that the American Pharmaceutical Association, in 1862, decided to abolish its Committee on Adulterations to avoid further attacks which the critics of the profession were directing against it as a whole because of the derelictions of individuals. The association, however, created a new Committee on the Drug Market that was charged among other duties with the responsibility of making an annual report of adulterations. *Proceedings of the American Pharmaceutical Association,* 1862, p. 28. For a list of adulterations, see Squibb, "Report on the Drug Market [1863]," pp. 177-192.

127. Squibb wrote in 1857: "It is abundantly demonstrated by daily experience that more chemical research and labor are now required to discriminate between good and bad medicinal substances, than for the proper preparation of most of them, while many, from their character, defy all proper scrutiny. For instance, it is far easier to make medicinal hydrocyanic acid, than to ascertain the strength or

purity of an unknown sample, while such substances as compound extract of colocynth can never have their value determined by examination. . . ." See Edward R. Squibb, "The Manufacture, Impurities, and Tests of Chloroform," AJP, Vol. 29 (September 1857), p. 431. As late as 1882, Squibb suggested a crude physiological method of standardization for aconite before an attempt was made to standardize it by its alkaloidal content. See Manuel G. Jauregui, "The Biological Assay of Aconite," *Journal of the American Pharmaceutical Association*, Vol. 16 (November 1927), p. 1046. See also, the interesting growth of assays of syrup of ferrous iodide, Caty J. Braford and H. A. Langenhan, "A Pharmaceutical Study of Syrup of Ferrous Iodide, 1840-1927," ibid. (July 1927), pp. 656-660.

128. On the great lack of uniformity in the products of the drug manufacturers see "Fluid Extracts," AJP, Vol. 30 (July 1858), pp. 382-383; "Chemical versus Pharmaceutical Manufacturers," *Druggists' Circular*, Vol. 9 (October 1865), p. 210.

129. *A Statement of the Causes Which Led to the Dismissal of Surgeon General William A. Hammond from the Army*, pp. 55-56.

130. Ibid., p. 56; Hammond to A. H. Reeder, President of the Special Commission of the War Department, July 22, 1863, Hammond court martial trial; Maxwell, *Lincoln's Fifth Wheel*, p. 85.

131. John M. Maisch, "Statistics of the U.S. Army Laboratory at Philadelphia," *Proceedings of the American Pharmaceutical Association*, 1866, p. 275; Robert Murray testimony, Hammond court martial trial.

132. See Squibb's price lists and printed circulars dated November 1859; May 1860; August 1, 1861; January 16, 1863; February 1, 1863; November 30, 1863; April 14, 1864; June 20, 1864; July 18, 1864; August 18, 1864; February 22, 1865; August 4, 1865. Squibb offered "discounts proportionate to the amounts sold," but abandoned that practice in January 1863. Price lists and circulars are in the Squibb Institute for Medical Research Library, New Brunswick, New Jersey.

133. "The Case of Surgeon-General Hammond," *Druggists' Circular*, Vol. 8 (August 1864), p. 168; Maxwell, *Lincoln's Fifth Wheel*, pp. 234-237.

134. [William Procter Jr.] "Editorial Department," AJP, Vol. 35 (May 1863), p. 283.

135. MSH, Part III, Vol. 1, p. 965.

136. Barnes to Stanton, September 19, 1863 (fair copy), SG Letterbooks, Letters to the Secretary of War; OR, Series III, Vol. 2, p. 752.

137. C. O. Whelan to James C. Dobbin, October 19, 1853 (fair copy); Edward H. Squibb to Charles F. Chandler, March 14, 1911; Captain D. W. Knox, United States Navy (retired) to Ira B. Tice, October 10, 1942, Squibb MSS; "The United States Naval Medical Depot," *United States Naval Medical Bulletin*, Vol. 11 (1917), pp. 337-342; "Overview: A Brief Account of Naval Medical Department Activities, 1775-1940," MS., in National Archives.

138. Hammond to Stanton, November 10, 1862 (fair copy), Surgeon General's Report Books.

139. "Affidavit of Surgeon J. R. Smith," July 26, 1879, Hammond ACP file, AGO.

140. A. K. Smith, Surgeon United States Army, to E. S. Dunster, Assistant Surgeon United States Army, September 14, 1863, SGO, Letters Received.

141. Moore to Stanton, November 3, 1862, SGO, Letters Received.

142. Stevens to Hammond, December 1, 1862, January 16, 1863, SGO, Letters Received.

143. Satterlee to id., February 3, 1863, SGO. Letters Received.

144. Stevens to Hammond, December 1, 1862, SGO, Letters Received.

145. Stevens organized Hennell Stevens and Company, Manufacturing and Analytical Chemists, in Philadelphia, after his graduation from the Philadelphia College of Pharmacy in the 1850s. The Stevens firm specialized in the production of glycerin by the steam process (he wrote his thesis on glycerin) and rare chemicals. Their price list, according to one contemporary notice, comprised over 200 different chemicals. His enterprise was succeeded, however, by Pascoe and Brother. See printed sales circular of Pascoe and Brother, August 1858, and the business card of Hennell Stevens & Co., both in SGO, Letters Received; full-page advertisement of Hennell Stevens & Co. in AJP, Vol. 31 (March 1859), advertising section, p. 15; Hennell Stevens, "Glycerin," AJP, Vol. 30 (January 1858), pp. 88-89. Edwin T. Freedley, *Philadelphia and Its Manufacturers* (Philadelphia, Edward Young, 1858), p. 209; Francis B. Heitman, *Historical Register and Dictionary of the United States Army from Its Organization, September 29, 1789, to March 2, 1903,* 2 vols. (Washington, Government Printing Office, 1903), Vol. 1, p. 922.

146. Creamer to Wood, January 5, 1863, SGO Letters Received.

147. Heitman, *Historical Register,* Vol. 1, p. 337.

148. Creamer to Hammond, October 28, 1862, SGO, Letters Received.

149. Id. to id., December 2, 1862, SGO, Letters Received.

150. Id. to Wood, January 5, 1863, SGO, Letters Received.

151. Alden, By Order of the Surgeon General, to Creamer, January 12, 1863 (fair copy), SG Letterbooks, Military Letters.

152. Id. to Wood, March 16, 1863 (fair copy, endorsement), SG Letterbooks, Military Letters.

153. Creamer to Hammond, March 10, 1863, SGO, Letters Received.

154. Creamer, "Statement of the Operations of the 'Work Room,' or 'Laboratory' Attached to the Medical Purveying Depot, Saint Louis, Mo. from its Commencement on the 1st of March 1863 to the 31st of July 1863," SGO, Letters Received.

155. Dunster, By Order of the Surgeon General, to Creamer, July 25, 1863 (fair copy), SG Letterbooks, Military Letters; Creamer to Hammond, July 30, 1863, SGO, Letters Received.

156. E. T. Whittingham, Assistant Surgeon U.S. Army, By Order of the Surgeon General, to Creamer, August 27, 1863 (fair copy), SG Letterbooks, Military Letters. Creamer was transferred to another post, but he was finally mustered out of the service with an honorable discharge in December 1865. See Heitman, *Historical Register,* Vol. 1, p. 337.

157. C. H. Crane, Surgeon U.S. Army, By Order of the Surgeon General, to id., December 8, 22, 1863 (fair copies), SG Letterbooks, Military Letters.

158. Hammond to Stanton, November 10, 1862 (fair copy), Surgeon General's Report Books.

Chapter 2

1. On the quarrel between Hammond and Stanton, see Louis C. Duncan, "The Strange Case of Surgeon General Hammond," *The Military Surgeon,* Vol. 64 (January-February 1929), p. 104.

2. Hammond further instructed Smith "to report to this office the price at which such buildings when found can be leased or purchased and the circumstances which have guided you in this connection. Reference may be had to the future adaptation of a steam engine." See J. R. Smith, By Order of the Surgeon General, to A. K. Smith July [sic January 1863], in Hammond court martial trial.

3. McCormick to Hammond, January 19, 1863 (telegram) SGO, Letters Received; Hammond to Satterlee, January 21, 1863, Hammond court martial trial. Hammond instructed Satterlee, "I design to detail Surgeon C. McCormick, U.S.A., on duty in the city of New York, connected with the Purveying Dept. of the Army. On receipt of order assigning him in this duty, I desire you to rent the building selected by him, for one year, with the privilege of a longer lease if desired by the Government, which he will be authorized to fit up as a laboratory for the preparation of such articles of medical and hospital supplies as can be economically prepared, and which may be further determined on. The detail of this arrangement will be hereafter communicated to you and Surg. McCormick."

4. Barnes to Meigs, October 15, 1863 (endorsement, fair copy), SG Letterbooks, Letters to the War Department.

5. Bill to Barnes, February 26, 1864; Printed Circular, John Hyer Jr., Manufacturing Chemist, Astoria, Long Island, both in SGO, Letters Received; Hammond to Meigs, April 20, 1863 (fair copy), SG Letterbooks, Letters to the War Department.

6. McCormick to Hammond, March 31, 1863, SGO Letters Received; E. S. Dunster, By Order of the Surgeon General, to Satterlee, April 4, 1863 (fair copy), SG Letterbooks, Military Letters.

7. A. K. Smith to id., January 24, 1863, Andrew K. Smith File, Personal Papers, Medical Officers and Physicians, AGO, War Department, National Archives, RG 94.

8. Hammond to Stanton, February 27, 1863 (fair copy), SG Letterbooks, Letters to the Secretary of War.

9. Barnes to id., September 17, 1863 (fair copy), SG Letterbooks, Letters to the Secretary of War; A. K. Smith to Dunster, September 14, 1863, SGO, Letters Received.

10. Id. to Hammond, January 19, 1863, SGO, Letters Received.

11. A. K. Smith to Murray, March 3, 1863 (copy), in Hammond court martial trial (testimony of Robert Murray).

12. Id. to Hammond, January 29, 1863, SGO, Letters Received.

13. Id. to id., January 24, 1863, Andrew K. Smith File, AGO.

14. John Maisch, "Statistics of the U.S. Army Laboratory at Philadelphia," *Proceedings of the American Pharmaceutical Association,* 1866, p. 273.

15. A. K. Smith to Hammond, January 19, 1863, SGO, Letters Received.

16. Id. to id., January 29, 1863, SGO, Letters Received.

17. Hammond to Meigs, February 2, 1863 (fair copy), SG Letterbooks, Letters to the War Department.

18. Quartermaster General Office, Register of Contracts, War Department, National Archives, RG 92.

19. Hammond to Meigs, February 12, 1863 (fair copy), SG Letterbooks. Letters to the War Department.

20. For a description of this building, see Edwin T. Freedley, *Philadelphia and Its Manufacturers,* (Philadelphia, Edward Young, 1858) p. 444. The hospital, known as the Master Street Hospital, was opened July 1, 1862 and continued in operation until the Chestnut Hill (Mower) Hospital was receiving patients. See Frank H. Taylor, *Philadelphia in the Civil War, 1861-1865* (Philadelphia, "Published by the City," 1913), p. 228.

21. A. K. Smith to Hammond, February 13, 1863, SGO, Letters Received.

22. C. C. Byrne, By Order of the Surgeon General, to W. T. King, U.S. Army Medical Director, Philadelphia, April 21, 1863 (fair copy), SG Letterbooks, Military Letters.

23. A. K. Smith to Hammond, April 13, 1863, SGO, Letters Received.

24. Ibid.

25. Maisch, "Statistics of the U.S. Army Laboratory," p. 273; Maisch declared that the operations in the laboratory began about April 15, and that two weeks later they were prepared to begin making deliveries. Maisch testimony, Hammond court martial trial.

26. Barnes to Stanton, September 19, 1863 (fair copy), SG Letterbooks, Letters to the Secretary of War.

27. Special Order No. 43, March 19, 1863, AGO, War Department; Letters of Instructions, Surgeon General's Office to A. K. Smith, March 12, 1863 (fair copy), SG Letterbooks, Military Letters.

28. Barnes to Stanton, September 17, 1863 (fair copy), SG Letterbooks, Letters to the Secretary of War.

29. J. R. Smith, By Order of the Surgeon General, to Satterlee, April 20, June 13, 1863; same to Murray (fair copies), SG Letterbooks, Military Letters.

30. Barnes to Stanton, September 19, 1863 (fair copy), SG Letterbooks, Letters to the Secretary of War.

31. "Requisition for apparatus required in the U.S. Med. Laboratory, Philadelphia from Surg. A. K. Smith, U.S.A., in charge, March 24, 1863," (endorsement by C. H. Alden, By Order of the Surgeon General, fair copy); J. B. Smith to A. K. Smith, March 12, 1863 (fair copy), SG Letterbooks, Military Letters.

32. After Hammond was no longer surgeon general, Murray, the medical purveyor at Philadelphia, wrote: ". . . It is proper to state that I was not consulted in any matters connected with the establishment of the Laboratory. . . . The late Surgeon General consulted only with Surgeon Smith as to what articles should be

prepared at the laboratory. . . . Under these circumstances I stated to the late Surgeon General that I considered my connection with the Laboratory as merely nominal & except when requested by Dr. Smith have not taken any control over it." See Murray to Barnes, September 2, 1864, SGO, Letters Received.

33. Stanton ordered the following endorsement to be written on Hammond's request to visit New York City: "In the opinion of the Secretary of War it is the duty of a Chief of Bureau to remain in Washington and transact his business by writing." Hammond to Stanton, March 2, 1863 (endorsement, fair copy), SG Letterbooks, Letters to the Secretary of War.

34. J. B. Smith, By Order of the Surgeon General, to McCormick (in care of Medical Purveyor, New York), April 14, 1863 (fair copy); same to A. K. Smith (in care of Medical Purveyor, Philadelphia); id. to id., April 21, 1863 (fair copy), SG Letterbooks, Military Letters. Hammond also ordered Andrew K. Smith to visit New York for discussions with McCormick.

35. A. K. Smith to Hammond, April 13, 1863, SGO, Letters Received. Joseph Janvier Woodward was born October 30, 1833; in 1853 he was a graduate in medicine from the University of Pennsylvania. After one year's residency at the Philadelphia Hospital, he taught surgery for a number of years at his alma mater until, in 1861, he passed the Army Medical Board examination. On June 9, 1862, Hammond directed him to take charge of the medical section of the medical and surgical history of the war, and the reports of sick and wounded soldiers for pension claims; about the same time he became administrator of the Army Medical Museum. He also made various "microscopal and chemical examinations" for the medical department; in these he often differed with the Philadelphia laboratory's staff over testing procedures. On Woodward, see Memoranda [undated and unsigned] and "Memorandum of the Military Services of J. J. Woodward, Assistant Surgeon U.S. Army," in Joseph Janvier Woodward File, Personal Papers, Medical Officers and Physicians, AGO, War Department, National Archives, RG 94; Woodward testimony, Hammond court martial trial.

36. J. R. Smith, By Order of the Surgeon General, to A. K. Smith, March 13, 1863 (fair copy), SG Letterbooks, Military Letters.

37. Alden, By Order of the Surgeon General, to id., March 12, 1863 (fair copy), SG Letterbooks, Military Letters.

38. Hammond to McCormick, April 20, 1863 (fair copy), SG Letterbooks, Military Letters.

39. A. K. Smith to Hammond, May 11, 1863, SGO, Letters Received.

40. Squibb to T. G. Catlin, February 16, 1863 (photostat), Squibb MSS.

41. Hammond to Stanton, October 18, 1862 (fair copy), SG Letterbooks, Letters to the Secretary of War.

42. Unlike Satterlee, Murray did not have close connections with the drug manufacturing industry. He came from Baltimore (Hammond's home city), belonged to a prominent family, was a graduate of the University of Pennsylvania, and had been known "from boyhood" by Chief Justice Roger B. Taney. As a young physician Murray was recommended for appointment by an Army Medical Board in 1844, and thereafter followed the usual career of an army medical offi-

cer—contract surgeon, assistant surgeon, and surgeon at various posts but most of the time in California until the outbreak of the Civil War. His father, Daniel Murray, was once a naval officer. After the Civil War, Murray received other promotions until his long service culminated in his appointment as surgeon general on February 9, 1884. He retired with the rank of Brigadier General, August 6, 1886. See File of Robert Murray, Personal Papers, Medical Officers and Physicians, Adjutant General's Office, War Department, National Archives, RG 94.

43. Murray to Barnes, September 2, 1864, SGO, Letters Received.

44. Maisch, "Statistics of the U.S. Army Laboratory," p. 273.

45. On Satterlee, see Richard S. Satterlee file, Personal Papers, Medical Officers and Physicians, AGO, War Department, National Archives, RG 94; James N. Phalen, "Richard Sherwood Satterlee," *Dictionary of American Biography,* Vol. 16 (New York, Scribner's, 1935), p. 376.

46. Ibid.

47. For Hennell Stevens' scheme, see Chapter 1.

48. Satterlee to Hammond, February 3, 1863, SGO, Letters Received. On the Satterlee Hospital, see Taylor, *Philadelphia in the Civil War,* p. 225 and illustration facing that page. Also, Winnifred K. MacKay, "Philadelphia During the Civil War, 1861-1865," *Pennsylvania Magazine of History and Biography,* Vol. 70 (January 1946), p. 25. It was known also as the West Philadelphia Hospital. See also, MSH, Part III, Vol. 1, p. 926.

49. Hammond was indiscreet when he wrote to Medical Purveyor George E. Cooper of Philadelphia: "How would you like to go to New York as Purveyor? I can't get Satterlee to take a sufficiently large view of the present emergency. He is a good old fellow but terribly slow. He does not seem to be able to comprehend the idea of an army of over 15,000 men or an expenduture of over 100,000 dollars a year." Hammond to Cooper, June 17, 1862 (fair copy), Hammond court martial trial.

50. On Satterlee's candidacy for the surgeon general's office, see Phalen, "Satterlee," p. 376; Louis C. Duncan, *The Medical Department in the Civil War* (n.p., no pub., n.d.), "Evolution of the Ambulance Corps and Field Hospital," p. 8. For a reference to the Satterlee Hospital in Philadelphia, see Victor Robinson, *White Caps: The Story of Nursing* (Philadelphia, J. B. Lippincott, 1946), p. 179.

51. Satterlee to Hammond, May 28, 1862, Richard S. Satterlee file, AGO. In this letter Satterlee wrote: "I desire to remind the Surgeon General, that while himself, many of the Medical officers, all the people employed in and about my office are much benefited by the new order of things, I am in comparison, with greatly increased labor and responsibility, where I was thirty years ago. Has any man been more faithful to the country; has any member of the medical profession done more to increase its usefulness, or to sustain its dignity and honor than myself? Is there anything in the medical service, or the duties of the Medical Purveyor, incompatible with reward for long and faithful service, or the benefit to be derived from the brevet rank and pay of a Brigadier General?"

52. Hammond to [Stanton], March 9, 1863 (fair copy), SG Letterbooks, Letters to the Secretary of War.

53. Frances B. Heitman, *Historical Register and Dictionary of the United States Army from Its Organization, September 29, 1789, to March 2, 1903*, 2 vols. (Washington, Government Printing Office, 1903), Vol. 1, p. 860.

54. J. R. Smith, By Order of the Surgeon General, to Satterlee, February 20, 1863 (fair copy); Hammond to id., March 4, 1863, both in SG Letterbooks, Military Letters.

55. Satterlee to Hammond, March 9, 1863, SGO, Letters Received.

56. Alden, By Order of the Surgeon General, to Satterlee, March 11, 1863 (fair copy), SG Letterbooks, Military Letters.

57. Satterlee to Hammond, March 14, 1863, SGO, Letters Received.

58. J. R. Smith, By Order of the Surgeon General, to Satterlee, March 16, 1863 (fair copy), SG Letterbooks, Military Letters.

59. Satterlee to Hammond, March 17, 1863, SGO, Letters Received. Satterlee wrote: "I trust that it is unnecessary I should assure the Surgeon-General, that whatever ability I possess, as it has been gained in the service of my country, in the Medical Corps of the Army—and therefore belongs to it, shall be cheerfully devoted to its best interests in the operations of the Laboratory."

60. Id. to id., March 9, 1863, SGO, Letters Received.

61. On these debts, see for example, Squibb to Hammond, March 24, 1863, SGO, Letters Received.

62. Satterlee to id., March 17, 1863, SGO, Letters Received.

63. Joseph P. Remington, "Edward Robinson Squibb, M.D.," AJP, Vol. 73 (September 1901), pp. 419-431; Andrew G. Du Mez, "Edward Robinson Squibb," *Dictionary of American Biography,* Vol. 17 (1935), p. 487.

64. "Editorial. Edward Robinson Squibb," AJP, Vol. 72 (December 1900), p. 600; Joseph P. Remington, "Memorial Address . . . ," *The Journal of E. R. Squibb, MD,* 2 vols. (n.p., privately printed, E. R. Squibb and Sons, 1930), Vol. 2, p. 630; Edward R. Squibb Circulars [Price Lists], May 1860 and November 30, 1863, Squibb MSS. Squibb wrote: ". . . The success achieved by this Laboratory, through the unwavering and determined support extended to it by the Army Medical Purveyor at New York prior to the establishment of the Army Laboratories, would be both undeserved and misplaced, if not used in the furtherance of these objects which alone obtained for it this support and patronage." From July 1 to December 31, 1862, Squibb was paid $63,460.22 for supplies that he sold to the medical department. "Summary statement of supplies purchased for the Medical and Hospital Department of the Army from July 1st, 1862 to December 31st, 1862," Hammond court martial trial.

65. Satterlee to Wright, [n.d.], Squibb MSS.

66. Frank Hastings Hamilton, *A Practical Treatise on Military Surgery* (New York, Blanchard & Lea, 1861).

67. *Brooklyn Daily Eagle,* December 30, 1858.

68. E. R. Squibb, Printed Form Letter [untitled], November 12, 1861, Squibb MSS; "A Lesson in Life," *Druggists' Circular,* Vol. 5 (Dec. 1861), p. 235; Lawrence G. Blochman, *Doctor Squibb* (New York, Simon and Schuster, 1958), pp. 134-135.

69. E. Kremers and G. Urdang, *History of Pharmacy* (Philadelphia, Lippincott, 1940), p. 318.

70. E. R. Squibb Time Book, Squibb MSS.

71. Joseph H. Bill, "Preliminary Report on the Arrangements and Operations of Dr. E. R. Squibb's Laboratory," March 9, 1863, SGO, Letters Received.

72. Squibb to Hammond, March 24, 1863, SGO, Letters Received; Murray, "Summary statement of medical supplies purchased . . ." Hammond court martial trial. According to this statement, Murray's office paid $10,958.31 to Squibb for panniers on February 16, 1863. Satterlee paid $33,207.00 to Squibb for panniers filled on March 19, 1863. See "Supplies bought by Richard S. Satterlee and paid for by him during the quarter ending June 30, 1863," SGO, Letters Received.

73. Squibb to Hammond, October 20, 1862, SGO, Letters Received; *Directions Concerning the Manner of Obtaining and Accounting for Medical and Hospital Supplies for the Army with a Standard Supply Table* (Washington, Government Printing Office, 1862), pp. 7-8. See also, Edward R. Squibb, Circular [Price List], February 1, 1863. Squibb's chlorine package contained "in a pasteboard box, a half gallon bottle of Sulphuric Acid Mixture, and 130 powders of a mixture of Common Salt and Binoxide of Manganese, with directions for use as a disinfectant." Squibb's contribution lay in his careful experimentation to establish the quantity which was effective to use as "a gaseous disinfectant" without being "hurtful or very disagreeable" to patients in hospitals and sick rooms.

74. As Squibb phrased it, the question was, more specifically, "on the comparative clinical effect of morphine trisulphate prepared from bleached and unbleached alkaloid." See Squibb to Austin Flint, May [n.d.] 1862, Squibb MSS.

75. An example of implied criticism outside the army perhaps may also be drawn from the "Report of a Committee of the Boston Society for Medical Improvement, On the Alleged Dangers Which Accompany the Inhalation of the Vapor of Sulphuric Ether," *Boston Medical and Surgical Journal,* Vol. 65 (October 24, 1861), p. 230.

76. Squibb to Hammond, October 20, 1862, SGO, Letters Received. See Hammond to George E. Cooper, Medical Purveyor, U.S.A., Philadelphia, August 11, 1862 (copy), Hammond court martial trial. Hammond wrote: "Hereafter Medicine Panniers and Hospital Knapsacks of patterns recently adopted by this office (and made by Jacob Dunton of 917 Market Street, Philadelphia) will be issued by the Medical Purveyors. The Medicine Panniers will supersede and be issued instead of Medicine Chests, they being so constructed as to be applicable for both. Requisitions for them will be made on Dr. George E. Cooper, Medical Purveyor, U.S.A. Philadelphia."

77. Dunster, By Order of the Surgeon General, to Murray, April 4, 1863 (fair copy), SG Letterbooks, Military Letters.

78. Squibb to Hammond, March 28, 1863, SGO, Letters Received.

79. The Medical Department did not discontinue the issue of Squibb's panniers entirely; when Joseph K. Barnes took over Hammond's duties he directed that they should be continued. Nevertheless, there were thirty-two employees on Squibb's payroll during March 1863, and but twenty-one in the week ending Oc-

tober 21, 1863. Both the number of employees and their rate of wages were higher in the summer of 1864 when Squibb was again filling orders for panniers and knapsacks. See Crane, By Order of the Surgeon General, to Murray, September 25, 1863 (fair copy), SG Letterbooks, Military Letters; E. R. Squibb Time Book.

80. Benjamin Butler, *Butler's Book: Autobiography and Personal Reminiscences of Major-General Benj. F. Butler* (Boston, A. M. Thayer & Co., 1892), p. 403. Butler wrote further of McCormick: "He gave me great confidence because he entirely approved of what I had done, and relieved me from the load of care and anxiety. . . . He was one of the truest friends I ever had" (ibid., p. 895).

81. Major Charles R. Greenleaf, "Military Services of Dr. Charles McCormick, late Assistant Surgeon and Surgeon U.S. Army . . . December 7, 1879" (letter press copy), Charles McCormick file, Personal Papers, Medical Officers and Physicians, AGO, War Department, RG 94.

82. Squibb to Dr. T. G. Catlin, February 16, 1863 (photostat), Squibb MSS. All the credit for sanitary measures in New Orleans should not be given to McCormick. Thomas Hewson Bache, U.S. Volunteers, was medical director in that city most of the first summer that federal troops were there.

83. Id. to Hammond, January 28, 1863, SGO, Letters Received.

84. J. R. Smith, By Order of the Surgeon General, to Squibb, May 8, 1863 (fair copy), SG Letterbooks, Military Letters.

85. Squibb to Hammond, May 7, 1863, SGO, Letters Received.

86. A. K. Smith to Hammond, January 24, 1863, Andrew K. Smith file, AGO.

87. Squibb to Hammond, February 2, 1863, SGO, Letters Received.

88. J. R. Smith, By Order of the Surgeon General, to J. Simpson, Medical Director, Baltimore, February 5, 1863 (fair copy), SG Letterbooks, Military Letters.

89. This report is printed in George Winston Smith, Ed., "The Squibb Laboratory in 1863," *Journal of the History of Medicine and Allied Sciences,* Vol. 13 (July 1958), pp. 382-394.

90. When he transmitted Bill's report on the Squibb laboratory to Hammond, Satterlee commended Bill for his "careful observation," and called Hammond's attention to Bill's data "for a correct estimate of the expense of preparing and working a laboratory of equal capacity." See Satterlee to Hammond, March 11, 1863, SGO, Letters Received.

91. Bill to id., March 30, 1863, SGO, Letters Received.

92. Dunster, By Order of the Surgeon General, to McCormick, April 21, 1863, SG Letterbooks, Military Letters.

93. McCormick to Satterlee, February 28, 1863, SGO, Letters Received.

94. Satterlee to Hammond, March 9, 1863, SGO, Letters Received.

95. Bill, "Preliminary Report," SGO, Letters Received.

96. Squibb to Catlin, February 16, 1863 (photostat), Squibb MSS; Lawrence Blochman, *Doctor Squibb: The Life and Times of a Rugged Idealist* (New York: Simon and Schuster, 1958), pp. 136-137.

97. McCormick to Satterlee, February 28, 1863, SGO, Letters Received.

98. Hyer Circular [printed], in SGO, Letters Received.

99. McCormick to Satterlee, March 21, 1863, SGO, Letters Received.

100. Bill to Barnes, February 26, 1864, SGO, Letters Received.

101. J. R. Smith, By Order of the Surgeon General, to McCormick, May 14, 1863 (fair copy), SG Letterbooks, Military Letters.

102. McCormick to Hammond, May 19, 1863. Charles McCormick file, AGO.

103. Hammond wrote as follows: "There can be but one opinion in regard to your course, and had you been a private physician you would have been placed beyond the pale of professional association. I cannot consent that the standard of professional ethics in the Med[.] Corps of the Army should be lower than that which [is] in force among our brethren of civil life. . . . There is but one standard of propriety and you have failed to come up to it. . . ." See Hammond to McCormick, May 23, 1863 (fair copy), SG Letterbooks, Military Letters.

104. Satterlee to Bill, May 26, 1863, File of Joseph H. Bill, Personal Papers, Medical Officers and Physicians, AGO, War Department, National Archives, RG 94.

105. Hammond to Stanton, June 9, 1863 (fair copy), SG Letterbooks, Letters to the Secretary of War.

106. Id. to id., July 1, 1863, SG Letterbooks, Letters to the Secretary of War; J. R. Smith, By Order of the Surgeon General, to McCormick, July 29, 1863 (fair copy), SG Letterbooks, Military Letters; Special Order 294, AGO, 1863.

107. McCormick to Hammond, May 19, 1863, Charles McCormick file, AGO.

108. Squibb to Catlin, February 16, 1863 (photostat), Squibb MSS.

109. Id. to A. K. Smith, June 8, 1863, SGO, Letters Received.

110. Ibid.

111. A. K. Smith to Hammond, June 11, 1863, SGO, Letters Received.

112. J. R. Smith, By Order of the Surgeon General, to A. K. Smith, June 12, 1863 (fair copy), SG Letterbooks. Military Letters.

Chapter 3

1. Satterlee to Bill, May 26, 1863, File of J. H. Bill, Personal Papers, Medical Officers and Physicians, AGO, War Department, National Archives, RG 94.

2. On Wurtz, see C. A. Browne, "Henry Wurtz," *Dictionary of American Biography,* Vol. 20 (1936), pp. 571-572; Henry Wurtz, "On the Composition of the Water of the Delaware River," AJP, Vol. 28 (September 1856), pp. 427-429 (esp. p. 428 on Bill's use of the microscope).

3. Joseph H. Bill personal file, AGO.

4. Ibid. Bill to Brevet Col. C. H. Magan, March 31, 1866, Joseph H. Bill, ACP file, AGO, RG 94.

5. A. K. Smith to Hammond, June 11, 1863, SGO, Letters Received.

6. Ibid.

7. Bill to Satterlee, February 26, 1864, SGO, Letters Received. After he had won his point and the Astoria laboratory had been operating for over a year, Bill admitted that the laboratory's "building and place . . . [were] unsuited to the purpose, being generally inconvenient and unnecessarily expensive." He then spoke

of the buildings at the Astoria depot as "a miserable collection of sheds." Id. to id., December 31, 1864, SGO, Letters Received.

8. J. R. Smith, By Order of the Surgeon General, to id., June 12, 1863 (fair copy), SG, Letterbooks, Military Letters.

9. Satterlee to Hammond, March 14, 1863, SGO, Letters Received. Satterlee wrote: "I think, — commencing at the beginning of the Supply Table, — we could purchase, and pulverize when necessary, and put up, for example: the Acacia Gum, the aloes, and such of roots, barks, seeds &c, as the supply-table calls for. The acids could be purchased in carboys, and put up in bottles as required. The Alcohol and possibly Whiskey and Wine could be selected in barrels and bottled. The Tinctures may be made, and put up in proper quantities. The preparations of Ammonia could be purchased in quantity, and divided into small bottles. If we have the apparatus, the Extracts, or a part of them, could be made up; and other such like operations could be carried on; and as [we] progress others more difficult might be undertaken."

10. Dunster, By Order of the Surgeon General, to Satterlee, June 20, July 1, 1863 (fair copies), SG Letterbooks, Military Letters.

11. J. R. Smith, By Order of the Surgeon General, to A. K. Smith, July 24, 1863 (fair copy), SG Letterbooks, Military Letters.

12. A. K. Smith to Hammond, August 5, 1863, SGO, Letters Received.

13. Bill to Satterlee, July 8, 1863, SGO, Letters Received.

14. A. K. Smith to Hammond, August 5, 1863, SGO, Letters Received.

15. Satterlee to id., May 9, 1863, SGO, Letters Received; J. R. Smith, By Order of the Surgeon General, to Satterlee, June 13, 1863, and id. to Murray, June 13, 1863 (fair copies), SG Letterbooks, Military Letters.

16. Bill to Satterlee, July 18, 1863, SGO, Letters Received.

17. Whittingham, By Order of the Surgeon General, to id., August 18, 1863 (fair copy), SG, Letterbooks, Military Letters.

18. Bill to Hammond, through Satterlee, August 24, 1863, SGO, Letters Received.

19. OR, Series III, Vol. 3, p. 1199. Hammond was relieved of his duties with the Surgeon General's Bureau, and ordered to establish his headquarters in the Department of the Gulf. Joseph R. Smith, his friend and subordinate who was temporarily assigned Hammond's duties in the surgeon general's office, correctly surmised that the move was "an effort to make him [Hammond] resign or to crush him. . . ." See J. R. Smith to A. P. Meylert, medical purveyor, Louisville, August 30, 1863, Hammond court martial trial. Hammond, however, carried out his inspection mission by visiting the Medical Department's installations at Hilton Head, Louisville, St. Louis, and other points in the West. See Hammond to Stanton, October 5, 1863 (telegram, copy), Stanton MSS, Library of Congress.

20. Whittingham, By Order of the Surgeon General, to Bill, August 26, 1863 (fair copy), SG Letterbooks, Military Letters.

21. Id. to Satterlee, August 27, 1863 (fair copy), SG Letterbooks, Military Letters.

22. J. R. Smith, By Order of the Surgeon General, to A. K. Smith, June 15, 1863 (fair copy), SG Letterbooks, Military Letters.

23. A. K. Smith to Hammond, August 11, 17, 1863, SGO, Letters Received. Smith insisted that this was done with Bill's consent, and that after the transfer three sets of chasers and bedstones still remained at Astoria. According to Smith, Bill did not have sufficient steam power to run more than those and his kettles.

24. Id. to id., July 18, 1863, SGO, Letters Received.

25. Bill to Barnes, November 12, 1863, Joseph H. Bill file, AGO.

26. Id. to Hammond, August 1, 1863, SGO, Register of Letters Received; J. R. Smith, By Order of the Surgeon General, to Bill, August 3, 1863 (fair copy), SG Letterbooks, Military Letters; Frank Marquand enlisted in the United States Army on March 10, 1859. The date of his appointment as a hospital steward was February 1, 1862, and he was honorably discharged when his term of service expired at Astoria, March 10, 1864. See Register of Hospital Stewards, U.S. Army, Appointed Under Act of Congress approved August 16, 1856, p. 166, MS. in Surgeon General's records, National Archives, RG 112.

27. Bill to Hammond, June 20, 1863, SGO, Register of Letters Received.

28. Id. to Satterlee, September 16, 1863, SGO, Letters Received.

29. Id. to Barnes, February 26, 1864, SGO, Letters Received.

30. Id. to Satterlee, September 16, 1863, SGO, Letters Received.

31. McCormick to Surgeon General's office (endorsement by Bill), December 4, 1863, SGO, Letters Received.

32. Crane, By Order of the Surgeon General, to Satterlee, March 31, 1864 (fair copy), SG Letterbooks, Military Letters.

33. Id. to id., July 18, 1864 (fair copy), SG Letterbooks, Military Letters.

34. Bill to Barnes, February 24, 1864, SGO, Letters Received.

35. For a description of a pill-rolling machine developed during the 1850s, see "Pharmaceutical Apparatus," AJP, Vol. 24 (October 1852), pp. 315-316. Also, "Lewis's Patent Pill Machine," AJP, Vol. 26 (March 1854), pp. 118-119. These machines consisted of a pair of rollers, each containing hemispheric indentations that were moved toward each other by cogs, turned by a crank. The pill mass was squeezed into spherical molds when the rollers meshed. The machine, however, was judged impractical by one competent observer as late as 1867, the difficulty being that the pills did not fall free from the cylinders, but stuck in the molds unless oil or other extraneous materials were added to the pill mass. See Ferris Bringhurst, "On Pill Machines," *Proceedings of the American Pharmaceutical Association,* 1867, pp. 375-376. For the hand roller made of wood and brass by Parrish, employed in the United States Army Laboratories to make "immense numbers of pills," see Edward Parrish, *Treatise on Pharmacy,* (Third Edition, Philadelphia, J. B. Lippincott, 1864), pp. 50-51, 801. There was also invented during the Civil War a machine operated by a crank or treadle for automatically counting, boxing, and pushing out on a platform "ready to be carried away" 36,000 packages of pills in a ten-hour day; it was operated by two men and could be used also for the packaging of percussion caps. See "Machine for Counting Pills," *Druggists' Circular,* Vol. 8 (September 1, 1864), p. 188. A machine for

compressing tablets was built by Jacob Dunton in 1864, but this was only in the experimental stage during the Civil War, and tablets produced by it were not placed on the market until 1869. See Joseph England, Ed., *The First Century of the Philadelphia College of Pharmacy* (Philadelphia, The College, 1922), p. 156. William R. Warner of Philadelphia began the manufacture of sugar-coated pills on a large scale in 1857. See Charles H. Lawall, " 'Pharmaceutical Firsts' in Phila-delphia," *Journal of the American Pharmaceutical Association,* Vol. 15 (August 1926), p. 722.

36. Bill to Barnes, February 24, 1864, SGO, Letters Received.

37. Ibid.

38. Id. to Satterlee, December 31, 1864, SGO, Letters Received.

39. Id. to Barnes, February 24, 1864, SGO, Letters Received.

40. Crane, By Order of the Surgeon General, to Satterlee, December 23, 1863 (endorsement, fair copy), SG Letterbooks, Military Letters.

41. Id. to id., April 5, 1864 (endorsement, fair copy), SG Letterbooks, Military Letters.

42. Bill to id., December 31, 1864. SGO, Letters Received.

43. Id. to Barnes, February 26, 1864, SGO, Letters Received.

44. Charles E. Sonnenberg, "Ointments and Cerates," *Druggists' Circular,* Vol. 38 (February 1894), p. 27.

45. Tabular report accompanying Bill to Barnes, February 26, 1864, SGO, Letters Received.

46. Ibid.

47. Ibid.

48. Satterlee to Barnes, February 13, 14, 1865, SGO, Register of Letters Received.

49. Crane, By Order of the Surgeon General, to Murray, November 29, 1864 (fair copy), SG Letterbooks, Military Letters.

50. Bill to Satterlee, December 31, 1864, SGO, Letters Received.

51. "The U.S. Army Laboratory at New York," AJP, Vol. 37 (May 1865), p. 234. On the partial continuation of operations at Astoria, see "Correspondence: Reorganization of the Medical Staff," *The Army and Navy Journal,* Vol. 2 (August 5, 1865), p. 790.

52. "The U.S. Army Laboratory at New York," p. 234.

53. Crane, By Order of the Surgeon General, to Satterlee, February 15, 1865 (fair copy), SG Letterbooks, Military Letters.

54. "The U.S. Army Laboratory at New York," p. 234.

Chapter 4

1. Dunster, By Order of the Surgeon General, to Murray, April 21, 1863 (fair copy), SG Letterbooks, Military Letters.

2. J. R. Smith, By Order of the Surgeon General, to id., August 7, 1863 (fair copy), SG Letterbooks, Military Letters; A. K. Smith to Dunster, September 14, 1863, SGO, Letters Received.

3. Ibid.

4. Id. to Hammond, July 18, 1863, SGO, Letters Received.

5. Robert Murray, "A Statement of Purchases of Drugs, Materials &c. to be Prepared for Issue at U.S. Laboratory, and of Apparatus, Repairs, Wages &c. for the Laboratory," September 30, 1863 (fair copy), SGO, Register of Letters Received. The specific payroll figures were: May 1, $341.81; May 30, $877.89; June 30, $1,463.82; July 31, $2,238.63; August 31, $3,387.13; September 30, $3,736.11. Total wages paid to September 30, $12,055.39.

6. Barnes to Stanton, September 17, 1863 (fair copy), SG Letterbooks, Letters to the Secretary of War.

7. Testimony of Andrew K. Smith, February 20, 1864, Hammond court martial trial.

8. Murray, "Statement of Purchases."

9. For mention of Pittsburgh as a bottle manufacturing center of the pharmaceutical industry, see John W. Ballard, "The Old-Time Drug Store," *Journal of the American Pharmaceutical Association,* Vol. 15 (July 1926), p. 575.

10. A. K. Smith to Hammond, July 18, 1863, SGO, Letters Received.

11. Id. to Dunster, September 14, 1863, SGO, Letters Received. Creamer's use of old bottles at his St. Louis laboratory apparently convinced Hammond that similar "economies" could be effected at the Philadelphia laboratory. A flood of worthless receptacles of every size and shape: battered tin cans, chipped and filthy jars and bottles, some bearing manufacturers' imprints, began to inundate the laboratory, sent in by surgeons and stewards in the hospitals, medical storekeepers, and others. The laboratory was obliged to clean them in a separate wooden building, known as the wash house, and attempted to use them again, although it always had on hand a sufficient supply of its own bottles, either new or used. It was not until the spring of 1864 that Smith was able to secure a release from the scrubbing and storage of cast-off receptacles. A. K. Smith to Murray, March 24, 1864 (and endorsement), SGO, Letters Received.

12. [William Procter Jr.] "Editorial Department," AJP, Vol. 35 (July 1863), p. 375.

13. Murray, "Statement of Purchases."

14. A. K. Smith to Murray, March 3, 1863 (fair copy), in Testimony of Robert Murray, Hammond court martial trial.

15. Testimony of John M. Maisch, Hammond court martial trial.

16. Barnes to Stanton, September 17, 1863 (fair copy), SG Letterbooks, Letters to the Secretary of War.

17. P. M. Ashburn, *A History of the Medical Department of the United States Army* (Boston, Houghton Mifflin, 1929), p. 86; Louis C. Duncan, "The Strange Case of Surgeon General Hammond," *The Military Surgeon,* Vol. 64 (January-February 1929), p. 108.

18. Barnes to Stanton, September 17, 1863 (fair copy), SG Letterbooks, Letters to the Secretary of War.

19. Id. to id., October 31, 1863 (fair copy), SG Report Book.

20. A. K. Smith to Hammond, August 17, 1863, SGO, Letters Received.

21. Id. to [Surgeon General's Office], December 10, 1863, SGO, Letters Received.

22. Ibid.

23. Id. to Hammond, August 11, 17, 1863, SGO, Letters Received.

24. Whittingham, Assistant Surgeon U.S. Army, By Order of the Surgeon General, to Murray (fair copy, endorsement on requisition of A. K. Smith), October 15, 1863, SG Letterbooks, Military Letters.

25. Crane, By Order of the Surgeon General, to Murray, January 14, 1864 (fair copy, endorsement), SG Letterbooks, Military Letters.

26. A. K. Smith to [G. W. Crawford] Secretary of War, May 12, 1849; Alexander Hosack to [n.n.], October 23, 1851; "Military History of Andrew K. Smith," Andrew K. Smith file. Personal papers, Military Officers and Physicians, AGO. Smith was seasoned before the war by service in scattered army posts; from June to August 1861 he accompanied regular army troops from Fort Randall to Fort Abercrombie, and from there to Washington. After about one year of wartime duty in the office of the medical director of the Army of the Potomac, he became medical director at Hagerstown during the Antietam campaign. Hammond then intended to appoint him medical purveyor in Philadelphia, but changed his mind at the last minute and instead made him Medical Director of Transportation in Philadelphia (Robert Murray received the medical purveyor's appointment) and a member of the Medical Examining Board at that city. His next appointment was that of director of the United States Army Laboratory in Philadelphia. Hammond believed that A. K. Smith possessed more "business capacity" than Murray. See Hammond to Stanton, October 18, 1862 (fair copy), Samuel Cooper testimony, Hammond court martial trial.

27. Charles Pleis of Philadelphia filed charges against Smith with the surgeon general's office in which he accused Smith of being a "libertine." Pleis' charges were sent to Murray, but no action was taken by the Medical Department. The Pleis name was prominently associated with pharmacy in Philadelphia. John M. Pleis Jr. was a wholesale drug dealer and Mathias Pleis was one of the founders of the Philadelphia College of Pharmacy. For the Pleis charges, see Crane, By Order of the Surgeon General, to Murray, November 21, 1863 (endorsement, fair copy), SG Letterbooks, Military Letters.

28. A. K. Smith to McDougall, January 11, 1865, SGO, Letters Received. Maisch later said that he had immediate charge "of the manufacture and preparation of medicines and chemicals manufactured" at the laboratory. Maisch affidavit, August 7, 1879, Hammond ACP file, 79, AGO, RG 94.

29. M. I. Wilbert, "John Michael Maisch, An Ideal Pharmacist," AJP, Vol. 75 (August 1903), p. 357; Frank H. Taylor, *Philadelphia in the Civil War, 1861-1865* (Philadelphia, "Published by the City," 1913), p. 236.

30. A. K. Smith to Hammond, July 18, 1863, AGO, Letters Received.

31. John Maisch, "Statistics of the U.S. Army Laboratory at Philadelphia," *Proceedings of the American Pharmaceutical Association,* 1866, p. 273.

32. These characterizations of Maisch were found in various unidentified newspaper clippings that contained statements made at the time of Maisch's death

in 1893. See Clipping Book, Maisch MSS, Philadelphia College of Pharmacy and Science Library, Philadelphia; "Minutes of Meeting of the Members of the College," AJP, Vol. 65 (November 1893), pp. 556-557. See also Photo 4.4.

33. Ibid.

34. Joseph P. Remington, "Prof. J. M. Maisch," AJP, Vol. 66 (January 1894), pp. 1-3.

35. Wilbert, "John Michael Maisch, An Ideal Pharmacist," p. 355.

36. See the following articles and others by Maisch. "Notes on the Fluid Extracts of Buchu, Cimicifuga, Serpentaria, and Valerian," AJP, Vol. 31 (July 1859), pp. 312-314; "An Expeditious Mode of Making Mercurial Ointment," AJP, Vol. 28 (March 1856), pp. 106-107; "Remarks on Some Pharmaceutical Preparations," AJP, Vol. 30 (January 1858), pp. 12-15.

37. Remington, "Prof. J. M. Maisch," p. 3.

38. George Urdang, "Edward Parrish—A Forgotten Pharmaceutical Reformer," *The American Journal of Pharmaceutical Education,* Vol. 14 (January 1950), p. 225.

39. See advertisement in *Druggists' Circular,* Vol. 4 (July 1860), p. 248. This advertisement follows:

MAISCH'S
CHEMICAL AND PHARMACEUTICAL
LABORATORY, PHILADELPHIA

The undersigned gives instruction in practical pharmacy in E. Parrish's School of Pharmacy. He likewise instructs beginners and students in practical and analytical chemistry, attends to Chemical Analysis of all kinds, and prepares to order *Rare Chemicals* not generally met with in commerce.

John M. Maisch
800 Arch St., Philadelphia

40. "Prof. John M. Maisch, Phar.D.," [unidentified clipping], in Clipping Book, Maisch MSS. Parrish acknowledged this assistance, see Edward Parrish, *Treatise on Pharmacy,* (Third Edition, Philadelphia, J. B. Lippincott, 1864), p. vi. Maisch's close friendship with Parrish continued after he left Parrish's school. In 1863, when Maisch wished to be considered for the chief chemist's position at the United States Army Laboratory, it was through Parrish that he made application to Smith. See John M. Maisch testimony, Hammond court martial trial.

41. Curt P. Wimmer, *The College of Pharmacy of the City of New York,* included in *Columbia University in 1904: A History* (Baltimore, Printed by Read-Taylor, 1929), p. 51. Maisch taught in a third-floor room, at Waverly Place and Washington Street.

42. For an outline-prospectus of the course which Maisch taught in 1861-1862, see ibid., p. 55. The class met for three lectures each week at 7 p.m., Monday, Wednesday, and Friday evenings. Maisch's introductory address at the New York College of Pharmacy was printed in *The American Medical Times,* Vol. 3 (November 2, 1861), pp. 292-295.

43. One of these articles was on military medicine. See John M. Maisch, "Styptics Upon the Battle-Field," *Druggists' Circular,* Vol. 6 (August 1862), p. 134.

44. Remington, "Prof. J. M. Maisch," p. 3.

45. Barnes to Stanton, September 19, 1863 (fair copy), SG Letterbooks, Letters to the Secretary of War.

46. Id. to id., May 6, 1864 (endorsement, fair copy), SG Letterbooks, Letters to the Secretary of War.

47. A. K. Smith to Barnes, December 10, 1864 (précis, fair copy), SGO, Register of Letters Received.

48. Murray to id., December 15, 1864, SGO, Letters Received.

49. A. K. Smith to McDougall, January 11, 1865 (and endorsements), SGO, Letters Received.

50. Barnes to Stanton, January 26, 1865 (endorsement, fair copy), SG Letterbooks, Letters to the Secretary of War.

51. Maisch, "Statistics of the U.S. Army Laboratory," p. 273.

52. Joseph England, Ed., *The First Century of the Philadelphia College of Pharmacy* (Philadelphia, The College, 1922), pp. 217-218. The author of this sketch wrote that Diehl was "one of the foremost research workers of the country . . ." and added, "He will be remembered in American Pharmacy long after many of his contemporaries have been forgotten." After his graduation from the Philadelphia College of Pharmacy, Diehl (then only twenty-two years of age) became Chief of Laboratory for John Wyeth and Brother. The Wyeths recommended him to Andrew K. Smith.

53. C. Lewis Diehl Jr., "United States Army Laboratory," AJP, Vol. 78 (December 1906), p. 561.

54. England, Ed., *First Century,* p. 472; "Henry H. Jacobs," Enlistment Papers, AGO, RG 94.

55. William J. Scott, of Philadelphia, enlisted, July 1, 1863, and soon after that reported to Smith at the laboratory, Hospital Stewards of the Army, p. 31, AGO, RG 94.

56. Possibly this was the Charles Cummings, a young Pennsylvania farmer, born in Roscommon County, Ireland, who enlisted at Harrisburg on November 2, 1863. His enlistment papers do not indicate that he was a hospital steward. There is no "Charles L. Cummings" among the enlistment papers of the hospital stewards in the National Archives.

57. "William H. Webb," Enlistment Papers, AGO, RG 94. Webb, however, attended the Philadelphia College of Pharmacy *after* the war and was a graduate in 1868.

58. A. K. Smith to Barnes, December 19, 1864, SGO, Register of Letters Received. It was Hartshorne who vouched for William A. Stephens of New York when that individual made a contract with the Medical Department to furnish blankets. This blanket procurement was one of the transactions brought against Hammond at his court martial.

59. "Augustus Henkel," Enlistment Papers, AGO, RG 94.

60. J. R. Smith, By Order of the Surgeon General, to Murray, September 1, 1863 (endorsement, fair copy), SG Letterbooks, Military Letters.

61. A. K. Smith to McDougall, January 11, 1865, SGO, Letters Received.

62. Barnes to Stanton, December 10, 1863 (fair copy), SG Letterbooks, Letters to the Secretary of War.

63. J. R. Smith, By Order of the Surgeon General, to Murray, September 1, 1863 (endorsement, fair copy), SG Letterbooks, Military Letters.

64. Id. to id., March 12, 1863 (fair copy), SG Letterbooks, Military Letters; Murray to Hammond, September 7, 1863, SGO, Letters Received.

65. C[harles] McDougall, Surgeon and Brevet. Col., Medical Purveyor, Philadelphia, to Barnes, January 31, 1865, SGO, Letters Received.

66. See note 147 for an explanation of this quarrel.

67. Crane, By Order of the Surgeon General, to Murray, May 30, 1864 (fair copy), SG Letterbooks. Military Letters.

68. Frederick A. Keffer graduated from the Philadelphia College of Pharmacy in 1860. As a surgeon in the United States Army he was stationed at Satterlee Hospital from October 11, 1862, to May 28, 1863; he then went to New Orleans where he was medical purveyor, and was relieved from his command in the Department of the Gulf to report to Murray in Philadelphia on October 10, 1864. See England, Ed., *First Century,* p. 471; "Frederick A. Keffer," ACP file, AGO, RG 94.

69. A. A. Lee, Assistant Surgeon, U.S. Army, By Order of the Surgeon General, to Murray, October 20, 1864 (fair copy), SG Letterbooks, Military Letters.

70. Crane, By Order of the Surgeon General, to A. K. Smith, December 1, 1865 (fair copy), SG Letterbooks, Military Letters.

71. Id. to Murray, January 5, 1865 (endorsement, fair copy), SG Letterbooks, Military Letters.

72. Barnes to Stanton, January 19, 1865 (fair copy), SG Letterbooks, Letters to the Secretary of War; id. to McDougall, January 24, 1865 (fair copy), SG Letterbooks, Military Letters.

73. McDougall to Barnes, January 11, 1865, SGO, Letters Received.

74. Barnes to Stanton, December 21, 1864 (fair copy), SG Letterbooks, Letters to the Secretary of War. McDougall was not ordered to replace Murray until December 30, 1864. See E. D. Townsend, Assistant Adjutant General, to McDougall, Special Orders No. 474 (extract, copy), AGO.

75. Charles McDougall was a native of Ohio. He received his appointment as assistant surgeon, United States Army in 1832 (during the Black Hawk War). His most notable service during the Civil War came after the Battle of Shiloh when he served as medical director of the Department of the Mississippi. He was an admirer of Satterlee and recommended him for the surgeon general's appointment. In 1862 he joined Satterlee in New York City as medical director of the Department of the East. See Charles McDougall file, Medical Officers and Physicians, AGO.

76. For descriptions of the Ellis laboratory, see Evan Tyson Ellis, "The Story of a Very Old Philadelphia Drugstore," AJP, Vol. 75 (February 1903), pp. 57-71; William Haynes, *American Chemical Industry,* 6 vols. (New York, Van Nostrand Company, Inc., 1945-1954), Vol. 1, p. 211.

77. Joseph P. Remington, "Edward Robinson Squibb, M.D.," AJP, Vol. 73 (September 1901), p. 422.

78. [William Procter Jr.] "Editorial Department," AJP, Vol. 35 (July 1863), pp. 373-374.

79. Diehl, "United States Army Laboratory," p. 561.

80. Procter, "Editorial Department," AJP, Vol. 35 (July 1863), p. 373.

81. Diehl, "United States Army Laboratory," p. 560. See Photo 4.1.

82. Procter, "Editorial Department," AJP, Vol. 35 (July 1863), p. 374.

83. Ibid.; Maisch, "Statistics of the U.S. Army Laboratory at Philadelphia," p. 274.

84. Ibid., p. 273.

85. Procter, "Editorial Department," AJP, Vol. 35 (July 1863), pp. 374-375; Diehl, "United States Army Laboratory," p. 573. A pharmacist, however, directed the compounding of the pill mass.

86. Procter, "Editorial Department," AJP, Vol. 35 (July 1863), p. 374.

87. A. K. Smith to Hammond, August 5, 1863; id. to Dunster, September 14, 1863; id. to Barnes, December 10, 1863, SGO, Letters Received. In December 1863, Murray received permission to add as many sewing machines to the laboratory's sewing department as he thought necessary. See Crane, By Order of the Surgeon General to Murray, December 5, 1863 (fair copy), SG Letterbooks, Military Letters.

88. Id. to id., December 12, 1863 (fair copy), SG Letterbooks, Military Letters.

89. William Maxwell, *Lincoln's Fifth Wheel: The Political History of the United States Sanitary Commission* (New York: Longmans, 1956), p. 79.

90. Maisch, "Statistics of the U.S. Army Laboratory," p. 273.

91. Procter, "Editorial Department," AJP, Vol. 35 (July 1863), p. 374.

92. Diehl, "United States Army Laboratory," p. 571.

93. The process is described in Parrish, *Treatise on Pharmacy,* Third Edition, p. 527.

94. Procter, "Editorial Department," AJP, Vol. 35 (July 1863), p. 375.

95. Diehl, "United States Army Laboratory," pp. 573-574.

96. Procter, "Editorial Department," AJP, Vol. 35 (July 1863), p. 375.

97. The description of these buildings was written from floor plans that were found in SGO, Letters Received.

98. Diehl, "United States Army Laboratory," p. 561; Procter, "Editorial Department," AJP, Vol. 35 (July 1863), p. 373. The arrangement of the boilers and engine seemed to be about the same as at the Squibb laboratory. There the boiler provided steam for both the engine and the steam laboratory processes; the boiler was fed by a small pump which returned the water from the steam pipes used to heat the building. See Smith, Ed., "The Squibb Laboratory in 1863," p. 393.

99. There were also smaller percolators made of tinned iron.

100. Procter, "Editorial Department," AJP, Vol. 35 (July 1863), p. 374.

101. Diehl, "United States Army Laboratory," p. 561.

102. Ibid. The condensing apparatus was located on a platform above the stills.

103. A. K. Smith to Hammond, May 1, 1863 (J. R. Smith, By Order of the Surgeon General endorsement, fair copy), SG Letterbooks, Military Letters.

104. J. R. Smith, By Order of the Surgeon General, to A. K. Smith, July 17, 1863 (fair copy), SG Letterbooks, Military Letters.

105. A. K. Smith to Barnes, December 14, 1863, SGO, Letters Received.

106. Procter, "Editorial Department," AJP, Vol. 35 (July 1863), p. 374.

107. Diehl, "United States Army Laboratory," p. 560.

108. Maisch, "Statistics of the U.S. Army Laboratory," p. 274.

109. Ibid.; Diehl, "United States Army Laboratory," pp. 563-564.

110. Ibid. See also p. 55.

111. Ibid., p. 249; Parrish, *Treatise on Pharmacy,* Third Edition, p. 249. The vinegar of squill was made of powdered squill and acetic acid in the percolators of the stillroom.

112. Diehl, "United States Army Laboratory," p. 571.

113. Ibid.

114. Ibid., p. 572; John Farre, *Manual of Materia Medica and Therapeutics* (Philadelphia: Lea, 1866), p. 297; Parrish, *Treatise on Pharmacy,* Third Edition, p. 763.

115. Procter, "Editorial Department," AJP, Vol. 35 (July 1863), p. 373.

116. Parrish, *Treatise on Pharmacy,* Third Edition, p. 549.

117. Diehl, "United States Army Laboratory," p. 571; William Procter Jr., "Remarks on Monsel's Persulphate of Iron," AJP, Vol. 31 (September 1859), pp. 403-407. Persulfate of iron was also thought to have therapeutic value as an ointment in the treatment of hemorrhoids. See "Persulphate of Iron in Hemorrhoids," *Druggists' Circular,* Vol. 8 (August 1864), p. 163.

118. Diehl, "United States Army Laboratory," p. 565; Parrish, *Treatise on Pharmacy,* Third Edition, p. 565.

119. Farre, *Manual of Materia Medica,* p. 130; Samuel Jackson, "On the Therapeutical Applications of the Permanganate of Potash, and of Ozone," *The American Journal of Medical Sciences,* cited in *Druggists' Circular,* Vol. 8 (February 1864), pp. 28-29; "Permanganate of Potash in Infecting Ulcers, Ozena, etc.," *Paris Medical Gazette and Medical and Surgical Reporter,* cited in ibid. (August 1864), p. 163; Edward R. Squibb, "Permanganate of Potassa," ibid. (September 1864), p. 179; Diehl, "United States Army Laboratory," p. 572. Other operations were necessary before the crystals could be obtained. After the mass cooled, it was pulverized, boiled in water, allowed to stand until the insoluble matter was precipitated, the fluid decanted, then boiled again with more water, again decanted and dilute sulfuric acid added, evaporated and cooled until the crystals formed, drained, boiled with more water, strained, cooled, and the crystals dried. Only 4,125 pints of potassium permanganate were issued by the Philadelphia laboratory, and no crystals. The crucible process differed somewhat from that of Bechamp. For Bechamp's process, see "Preparation of Permanganate of Potassa," *Druggists' Circular,* Vol. 5 (January 1861), p. 59. Squibb's suggestion to improve

the Bechamp process by applying steam to the heated mass is in ibid., Vol. 8 (September 1864), p. 179.

120. Farre, *Manual of Materia Medica,* pp. 573-575; USD, Eleventh Edition, 1858, p. 841.

121. Diehl, "United States Army Laboratory," pp. 556-568. See also Photo 4.6.

122. Ibid., p. 572; Parrish, *Treatise on Pharmacy,* Third Edition, p. 435; Farre, *Manual of Materia Medica,* pp. 254-256.

123. C. Lewis Diehl Jr., "Remarks on Some Chemical Processes," *Proceedings of the American Pharmaceutical Association,* 1866, pp. 248-249.

124. Diehl, "United States Army Laboratory," pp. 568-571; Parrish, *Treatise on Pharmacy,* Third Edition, pp. 537-538; Edward R. Squibb, "Oleum Aethereum and Spiritus Aetheris Compositus," AJP, Vol. 29 (May 1857), pp. 193-204; J. M. Maisch, "On the Preparation of Heavy Oil of Wine," AJP, Vol. 37 (March 1865), pp. 101-105. Hoffmann's anodyne was prepared by mixing oleum aethereum with alcohol and ether. It was one preparation that almost never was made commercially by the officinal formula. In analyzing four commercial samples Procter found that all of them were deficient in heavy oil of wine. See Parrish, *Treatise on Pharmacy,* Third Edition, p. 538.

125. Ibid., p. 571.

126. Ibid., pp. 496-497; Farre, *Manual of Materia Medica,* pp. 793-794; Diehl, "United States Army Laboratory," p. 572.

127. The procedure followed in making silver nitrate was to take silver (in small pieces), mix it with nitric acid and distilled water, heat the solution on a sand bath, decant the clear solution into a porcelain capsule, evaporate half of it, and permit crystals to form. USD, Eleventh Edition, 1858, p. 945.

128. Diehl, "United States Army Laboratory," p. 565.

129. Dunster, By Order of the Surgeon General, to Murray, August 8, 1863 (endorsement, fair copy), SG Letterbooks, Military Letters; A. K. Smith to Hammond, June 10, 1863, SGO, Letters Received. This communication enclosed a bill from Balliere and Brothers and Westermann for books purchased, which had already arrived at the laboratory.

130. John M. Maisch, "Gleanings from German Journals," AJP, Vol. 36 (March 1864), pp. 107-113.

131. John M. Maisch, "On the Preparation of Heavy Oil of Wine," pp. 101-105. Squibb's formula is in his Notebook No. 6, Squibb MSS. See also, Edward R. Squibb, "Oleum Aethereum and Spiritus Aetheris Compositus," pp. 193-204. Squibb's formula was essentially the same as that given in the *United States Pharmacopoeia.* See USP, Fourth Decennial Revision, 1863, pp. 88-89. See also, Diehl, "Practical Observations on the Manufacture of Oleum Aethereum," *Proceedings of the American Pharmaceutical Association,* 1864, pp. 309-316.

132. Procter, "Editorial Department," AJP, Vol. 35 (July 1863), p. 373.

133. William C. Bakes, "Preparation and Dispensing of Plasters," *Proceedings of the American Pharmaceutical Association,* 1864, pp. 232-233. There is an illustration of Maisch's frame on p. 233.

134. Parrish, *A Treatise on Pharmacy,* Third Edition, p. 450.

135. Diehl, "United States Army Laboratory," pp. 566-568. For the use of condensers in processing quicksilver, see W. S. W. Raschenberger, "Notes on the Mercury of New Almaden, California," AJP, Vol. 28 (March 1856), pp. 97-101.

136. John M. Maisch, "Practical and Scientific Notes," AJP, Vol. 36 (March 1864), pp. 97-100.

137. Affidavit of Harrison Smith, August 12, 1879, Hammond ACP file, AGO; J. R. Smith, By Order of the Surgeon General, to Murray, August 26, 1863 (fair copy), SG Letterbooks, Military Letters; Murray to Hammond, August 28, 1863, SGO, Letters Received. From the letter last cited it is apparent that instead of forcing Harrison Smith upon the laboratory, Hammond was somewhat surprised, even critical, that Murray had engaged a drug broker to purchase crude drugs.

138. Murray, "A Statement of Purchases."

139. Murray to Barnes, March 7, 1864, SGO, Letters Received.

140. Crane, By Order of the Surgeon General, to Murray (fair copy), November 18, 1863; Dunster, By Order of the Surgeon General, to A. K. Smith (fair copy), June 10, 1863; Id. to H. N. Rittenhouse (fair copy), June 10, 1863; W. C. Spencer, By Order of the Surgeon General, to C. C. Cox (fair copy), January 29, 1864, SG Letterbooks, Military Letters; Murray testimony, February 9, 1864, Hammond court martial trial.

141. A. K. Smith to Dunster, September 14, 1863, SGO, Letters Received.

142. *Proceedings of the American Pharmaceutical Association,* 1862, p. 41.

143. USD, Eleventh Edition, 1858, p. 610.

144. George Graham to William J. M. Gordon, April 12, 1862, quoted in *Proceedings of the American Pharmaceutical Association,* 1862, pp. 227-228.

145. "Report of the Corresponding Secretary," ibid., 1863, pp. 172-173; Parrish, *Treatise on Pharmacy,* Third Edition, p. 383. There was also an opinion that American tartar contained too much tartrate of lime to make it fit for medical use as refined tartar, although it could be used in making tartaric acid. See USD, Eleventh Edition, 1858, p. 610.

146. J. R. Smith, By Order of the Surgeon General, to Murray, July 24, 1863 (fair copy), SG Letterbooks, Military Letters.

147. Murray to Hammond, August 9, 1863 (fair copy), Hammond court martial trial. Later, after relations between Murray and Andrew K. Smith had become somewhat strained, Murray intimated that Smith attempted to appropriate the authority to order samples directly from the dealers, and to decide for himself what wines and liquors would be bought for bottling at the laboratory. Murray further implied that in doing this Smith intended to extend favors to certain merchants. Hammond, however, assured Murray that he was mistaken if he believed that the surgeon general desired to have him patronize any particular dealer. In an amazingly unfair ruling during the Hammond court martial trial, Judge Advocate-General Joseph Halt held that because Hammond had ordered the medical purveyor to purchase no drugs or liquors without their prior testing at the laboratory, that Hammond conferred upon Smith, the director of the laboratory, supervision over

the purchase of all drugs and liquors tested. Speaking in his own defense, Hammond insisted that Smith had always been subordinate to the Philadelphia medical purveyor, and that no authority to purchase drugs or liquors as the surgeon general's personal agent had ever been given to Smith. If Smith ever had ambitions to control liquor purchases he quickly surrendered them; he merely reported to Murray on "the relative quality and price of the various samples inspected." Maisch could and did reject certain drugs which were found to be adulterated or below his minimum standards. See Murray testimony, February 10, 1864; Murray to Hammond, August 9, 1863 (fair copy), ibid; A. K. Smith to Dunster, September 14, 1863, SGO, Letters Received.

148. Maisch to A. K. Smith, January 13, 1865, Maisch MSS.

149. J. R. Smith to Stanton, June 5, 1863 (fair copy), SG Letterbooks, Letters to the Secretary of War; John M. Maisch, "Examinations of Brandy and Whiskey," *Proceedings of the American Pharmaceutical Association,* 1866, p. 268. For Molnar's description of his test, see M. Molnar, "Examination of Alcoholic Liquors to Ascertain Their Origin," AJP, Vol. 30 (May 1858), p. 273. One of the simple chemical tests used to detect copper in brandy was to add drops of olive oil to a sample of the brandy; after the sample was agitated and allowed to stand, the oil, when it separated, would have a greenish color. See "Means of Detecting and Separating Copper from Brandy," AJP, Vol. 26 (January 1854), pp. 86-87.

150. Maisch, "Examination of Brandy and Whiskey," pp. 267-269; Maisch to A. K. Smith, January 13, 1865, Maisch MSS. For tests developed after the Civil War that employed the Duboscq colorimeter, see E. Mohler, "Analysis of Brandy and Alcohol," AJP, Vol. 63 (July 1891), pp. 358-359.

151. John M. Maisch, "Assays of Sherry Wine," *Proceedings of the American Pharmaceutical Association,* 1866, pp. 269-272.

152. "Obituary. Prof. John M. Maisch," *Druggists' Circular,* Vol. 37 (October 1893), p. 238; see also, John M. Maisch, "On the Detection of Volatile Oils," *Proceedings of the American Pharmaceutical Association,* 1858, pp. 344-368.

153. "Minutes of the Fourteenth Annual Meeting," *Proceedings of the American Pharmaceutical Association,* 1866, p. 57. See also, "Minutes of the Pharmaceutical Meeting," AJP, Vol. 64 (April 1892), p. 217. In the last year of his life he still expressed the opinion "that the demand for good articles at fair prices would bring good articles, and that the success of the sale of poor articles was largely due to the demand for articles cheaper than they can be honestly produced."

154. John M. Maisch, "Report on the Drug Market," *Proceedings of the American Pharmaceutical Association,* 1864, p. 189.

155. Ibid., p. 188.

156. "Minutes of the Thirteenth Annual Meeting," ibid., 1865, p. 54.

157. John M. Maisch, "Impurities and Adulterations Noticed at the U.S. Army Laboratory, Philadelphia," AJP, Vol. 36 (March 1864), pp. 100-103.

158. Thomas Antisell, "Cultivation of the Cinchona in the United States," *Report of the Commissioner of Agriculture for the Year 1866,* p. 455.

159. Farre, *Manual of Materia Medica,* p. 636.

160. "Discoverers of Quinine," *Druggists' Circular,* Vol. 37 (October 1893), p. 229; James Grier, *A History of Pharmacy* . . . (London, The Pharmaceutical Press, 1937), p. 103.

161. John B. Biddle, *Materia Medica for the Use of Students* (Second Edition, Philadelphia, Lindsey and Blakiston, 1865), pp. 102-105; Parrish, *Treatise on Pharmacy,* Third Edition, p. 642.

162. "Philadelphia Correspondence," *Druggists' Circular,* Vol. 1 (October 1857), p. 137. This reporter wrote: "It is remarkable that the fluctuations in the price of this staple of our trade are never the direct result of advances or reductions in price made by the manufacturers, but arise from the increased demands upon holders and the consequent advance of the article in their hands. There is seldom a season when quinine may not be bought at a moderate price in the early summer; but if the autumn proves sickly as it advances, the price . . . experiences sometimes a rapid and enormous rise."

163. Adolph C. Meyers, *The Earlier Years of the Drug and Allied Trades in the Mississippi Valley* (St. Louis, privately printed, 1948), p. 151.

164. John W. Churchman, "The Use of Quinine During the Civil War," *Johns Hopkins Bulletin,* Vol. 17 (June 1906), p. 180; Churchman, however, exaggerated the rise in the price of quinine. See also, Squibb, "Report on the Drug Market," p. 182; M. L. Duran-Reynals, *The Fever-Bark Tree* (Garden City, New York, Doubleday & Company, Inc., 1946), p. 215.

165. J. R. Smith, By Order of the Surgeon General, to Murray, April 2, 1863 (fair copy), SG Letterbooks, Military Letters.

166. Alden, By Order of the Surgeon General, to Satterlee, March 28, 1863 (fair copy), SG Letterbooks, Military Letters.

167. A. K. Smith to Hammond, April 13, 1863, SGO, Letters Received.

168. *The New York Times,* April 1, 1863.

169. George E. Cooper, however, implied in his testimony at the Hammond trial that Hammond may have wished to give an advantage to John Wyeth and Brother, since Hammond ordered him to buy from the Wyeths sulfate of cinchonia manufactured by Powers & Weightman. See Cooper testimony, February 2, 1864, Hammond court martial trial.

170. Hammond to Murray, April 2, 1863 (fair copy), SG Letterbooks, Military Letters.

171. Testimony of Murray, February 11, 1864, Hammond court martial trial.

172. J. R. Smith, By Order of the Surgeon General, to Murray, March 12, 1863 (fair copy), SG Letterbooks, Military Letters. Italics not in original.

173. "The Quinine Sulfate Problem at the Philadelphia Laboratory," a transcript of a manuscript report dated April 17, 1863, from John M. Maisch to Andrew K. Smith, concerning a proposal to attempt the manufacture of quinine sulfate at the United States Army Laboratory, Philadelphia, was available on microfilm in 1962. It is now out of print.

174. Procter, "Editorial Department," AJP, Vol. 35 (July 1863), p. 375.

175. Alden, By Order of the Surgeon General, to Satterlee, June 13, 1862 (fair copy), SG Letterbooks, Military Letters.

176. Satterlee to Hammond, May 7, 23, 24, 1863 (précis, copy), SGO, Register of Letters Received.

177. Id. to id., March 26, 1863, SGO, Letters Received. In March 1863, for example, Rosengarten and Sons offered hospital quinine to Satterlee in five-ounce tins at $2.12½ per ounce; at that time Satterlee was paying $3.30 for bleached quinine sulfate.

178. Squibb, "Report on the Drug Market," p. 183.

179. Louis Pasteur, "On the Alkaloids of the Cinchonas," *AJP*, Vol. 25 (November 1853), p. 536; Wolfgang Felix von Oettingen, *The Therapeutic Agents of the Quiniline Group* (New York, The Chemical Catalogue Company, 1933), p. 125; Grier, *A History of Pharmacy*, p. 103; Parrish, *Treatise on Pharmacy*, Third Edition, pp. 642-649; Farre, *Manual of Materia Medica*, pp. 631-633. Very little was done with some of these alkaloids. See the statement in Farre, p. 631: "Quinia, quinidia, and cinchonia are the only alkaloids with whose operations we are acquainted." Pasteur designated the four principal alkaloids as quinine [quinia], quinidine [quinidia], cinchonine [cinchonia], and cinchonidine [cinchonidia]. Quinidine [quinidia] was isomeric with quinine [quinia].

180. "Philadelphia Correspondence," *Druggists' Circular,* Vol. 1 (October 1857), p. 137.

181. Squibb, "Report on the Drug Market," pp. 182-183; Haynes, *American Chemical Industry,* Vol. 1, p. 213. Hammond also directed Medical Purveyor George E. Cooper to purchase at least 120,000 ounces of cinchonia sulfate in the summer of 1862 although it was not yet on the supply table. See George E. Cooper testimony, February 2, 1864, Hammond court martial trial.

182. Maisch, "Report on the Drug Market," p. 196.

183. Parrish, *Treatise on Pharmacy,* Third Edition, p. 649.

184. Duran-Reynals, *The Fever-Bark Tree,* p. 185.

185. Van Oettingen, *Quiniline Group,* p. 135. These findings were not made public until 1867-1868.

186. Parrish, *Treatise on Pharmacy,* Third Edition, p. 649. The evidence from abroad was conflicting. See Farre, *Manual of Materia Medica,* p. 632; W. F. Daniell called it a failure after he tested cinchonia sulfate in West Africa, but J. E. Howard reported that it was used successfully in the East Indies. See Ferdinand F. Mayer, "Report on the Progress of Pharmacy," *Proceedings of the American Pharmaceutical Association,* 1863, pp. 106-107.

187. USP, Fourth Decennial Revision, 1863, p. 124.

188. Parrish, *Treatise on Pharmacy,* Third Edition, p. 649.

Chapter 5

1. "Report of the Secretary of War," *House Executive Documents,* Vol. 3, part 1, 39th Congress, 1st Session, pp. 24-25, 35.

2. Ibid., p. 35.

3. A. K. Smith to McDougall, May 2, 1865, SGO, Letters Received.

4. Bill to Satterlee, December 31, 1864, SGO, Letters Received. This report, according to regular procedure, was addressed to his immediate superior, Satter-

lee. But Bill knew, of course, that it would be sent to the surgeon general's office from New York City.

5. McDougall to [Surgeon General's Office], June 17, 1865, SGO, Letters Received.

6. Spencer, By Order of the Surgeon General, to McDougall, June 9, 1865 (endorsement, fair copy), SG Letterbooks, Military Letters.

7. Id. to Satterlee, March 7, 31, 1866 (fair copies); id. to McDougall, March 7, 1866 (fair copy), SG Letterbooks, Military Letters. Surgeon B. F. Bache, Director of the United States Navy Laboratory, New York, receipted for $23,422.43 of these medical supplies.

8. According to the surgeon general "most of the articles . . . [brought] their full value, and in some instances their cost price" at these sales. See "Report of the Secretary of War," 1865, p. 35.

9. *Catalogue of United States Sale: Drugs, Medicines, Instruments &c. to Be Sold at Auction on Friday Morning, August 4th, 1865, . . . By Samuel C. Cook, Auctioneer* ([Philadelphia], W. B. Selheimer Book and Job Printer [1865]), p. 11.

10. J. S. Billings, Assistant Surgeon, U.S. Army, By Order of the Surgeon General, to McDougall, November 21, 1865 (endorsement, fair copy); Spencer, By Order of the Surgeon General, to id., February 23; March 5, 15, 31; April 9, 1866 (endorsement, fair copies), SG Letterbooks, Military Letters.

11. A. K. Smith to McDougall, August 5, 1865, SGO, Letters Received.

12. "Report of the Secretary of War, 1865," p. 35.

13. Spencer, By Order of the Surgeon General, to Bill, November 11, 1865 (fair copy), SG Letterbooks, Military Letters.

14. Bill to Barnes, December 30, 1865, File of J. H. Bill, Personal Papers, Medical Officers and Physicians, AGO.

15. A. K. Smith to id., August 1, 1865, SGO, Letters Received.

16. Crane, By Order of the Surgeon General, to McDougall, October 23, 1865 (fair copy), SG Letterbooks, Military Letters.

17. Barnes to Stanton, November 23, 1865 (fair copy), SG Letterbooks, Letters to the Secretary of War; Spencer, By Order of the Surgeon General to Satterlee, December 2, 1865 (endorsement, fair copy), SG Letterbooks, Military Letters.

18. Bill to McDougall, March 29, 1866, SGO, Letters Received.

19. McDougall to Billings, November 12, 1867, SGO, Letters Received.

20. Ibid.

21. Id. to Barnes, January 20, February 18, 1868, SGO, Letters Received.

22. Bill to id., April 30, May 12, 26, 1868, File of J. H. Bill, Personal Papers, Medical Officers and Physicians, AGO.

23. McDougall to id., June 27, 1868, SGO, Letters Received.

24. Barnes to Stanton, September 19, 1863 (fair copy), SG Letterbooks, Letters to the Secretary of War.

25. See Bill to Satterlee, December 31, 1864, SGO, Letters Received. Bill was unfair to such reputable manufacturers as Squibb, but, however questionable his assumptions, his sincerity can scarcely be doubted in the following statement: "But the savings of this establishment [Astoria laboratory] is not its great advan-

tage. I think I may assert that it furnishes a *sufficient* supply of *reliable* medicines. This is the great advantage. . . . On *a priori* grounds it might be inferred that government could obtain by manufacture much better medicine than it could buy. I do not claim that officers of the army are more honest than civilians. This is not a question of honesty but of policy. It is the interest of a civilian to furnish as poor an article as possible for a given sum because his object is to make money. On the other hand it is the interest of an officer in charge of an arsenal or establishment of this kind to furnish as excellent an article as possible. His reputation is involved and this will be damaged if he issues a poor preparation."

26. McCormick to Barnes, June 6, 1864, SGO, Letters Received.

27. Maisch to A. K. Smith, July 18, 1865, SGO, Letters Received. On the insufficiency of chloroform at Gettysburg, see Testimony of F. Scott Bradner, Chaplain, 124th New York Volunteers, February 13, 1864, Hammond court martial trial.

28. Spencer, By Order of the Surgeon General, to McDougall, May 22, 1865 (fair copy), SG Letterbooks, Military Letters.

29. Id. to id., July 25, 1865 (fair copy), SG Letterbooks, Military Letters.

30. Id. to id., July 6, 1865 (fair copy), SG Letterbooks, Military Letters. This letter also stated that the medical purveyor in Washington was going to return to the Philadelphia purveyor all chloroform in his possession that had been made in Philadelphia.

31. Maisch to A. K. Smith, July 18, 1865, SGO, Letters Received.

32. Ibid.

33. Id. to id., August 29, 1865, Maisch MSS. See also, John M. Maisch, "The Specific Gravity of Medicinal Chloroform," *Proceedings of the American Pharmaceutical Association,* 1866, pp. 264-267.

34. Florence Yaple, "Pharmaceutical Meeting," AJP, Vol. 78 (April 1906), p. 202. Professor Joseph P. Remington recalled Squibb's wartime experience. See also, Edward Squibb, "The Manufacture, Impurities, and Test of Chloroform," AJP, Vol. 29 (September 1857), pp. 430-441.

35. David Brown, "Observations on Decomposing Chloroform," AJP, Vol. 65 (May 1893), pp. 241-244; Carl Schact and E. Blitz, "The Decomposition of Chloroform," *Pharmaceutical Journal and Transactions,* June 10, 1863, p. 1005, cited in AJP (July 1893), pp. 354-359.

36. During the Civil War, Thomas Antisell was Brigade Surgeon of Volunteers, Medical Director of the 12th Army Corps (Army of the Potomac), and Surgeon-in-Charge of Harewood Hospital. For these services he was brevetted colonel. He was also, in civilian life, Professor of Chemistry and Toxicology in Georgetown University Medical School; his title was later changed to Professor of Military Surgery, Physiology, and Hygiene. From 1866 to 1871, in addition to his duties at Georgetown, he was Chief Chemist of the United States Department of Agriculture. See A. Hunter Dupree, *Science in the Federal Government* (Cambridge, Massachusetts, The Belknap Press of Harvard University, 1957), pp. 152-153; "Thomas Antisell," *The National Cyclopaedia of America Biography* (1926 ed., New York, James T. White & Company, 1926), Vol. 19, pp. 448-449.

37. Crane, By Order of the Surgeon General, to A. K. Smith, May 16, 1864 (endorsement, fair copy), SG Letterbooks, Military Letters; Antisell to Barnes, May 15, 1864, SGO, Letters Received.

38. A. K. Smith to Murray, May 18, 1864, SGO, Letters Received.

39. Id. to Barnes, June 23, 1864 (and six enclosures), SGO, Letters Received.

40. John L. LeConte, Medical Inspector, Philadelphia, to A. K. Smith, May 18, 1864, SGO, Letters Received.

41. John M. Maisch, "On Some Medicinal Spirits," *Proceedings of the American Pharmaceutical Association,* 1864, pp. 303-308.

42. Such, however, was not the case. See USP (Fifth Decennial Revision, Philadelphia, J. P. Lippincott & Co., 1873), p. 277.

43. Squibb and Meyer to the Executive Committee of the American Pharmaceutical Association, November 10, 1864, in *Proceedings of the American Pharmaceutical Association,* 1864, pp. 54-55.

44. William Procter Jr., "The Officinal Fluid Extracts," AJP, Vol. 37 (May 1865), p. 182.

45. "Minutes of the Thirteenth Annual Meeting." *Proceedings of the American Pharmaceutical Association,* 1865, pp. 62-64.

46. Maisch's specific directions were: "Dissolve the carbonate of soda in twelve gallons of water, pour the solution into a still, add the alcohol, oil of lemon, nutmegs and lavender flowers, and macerate over night. Dissolve the muriate of ammonia in eight gallons of water, and after distillation has commenced, run the solution slowly, by means of a glass siphon, through the tubulus of the still head to near the bottom of the still. Apply heat and condense the distillate in a glass condenser, the discharge pipe of which reaches to near the bottom of the receiving vessel, and is afterwards kept below the surface of the distillate, of which forty gallons are obtained." Maisch, "On Some Medicinal Spirits," p. 308.

47. "Minutes of the Thirteenth Annual Meeting," 1865, p. 61. With this debate probably in mind, a pharmacists' journal carried an article that made the following commentary: "The rule of adhering strictly to the process of the pharmacopoeia comes under examination. Some look for uniformity by this means, and there can be no doubt of its value in such operations. The preparations are directed to be made in certain quantities in a certain way. But suppose the quantities multiplied by one hundred or one thousand, the apparatus constantly varying and improved, and the experience of the manufacturer supplying many added improvements in manipulation, perfecting the product, and economising material and labor—are these to be ignored?" See "Chemical versus Pharmaceutical Manufacturers," *Druggists' Circular,* Vol. 9 (October 1865), p. 210.

48. Diehl, "United States Army Laboratory," AJP, Vol. 78 (December 1906), p. 572.

49. Maisch to A. K. Smith, July 18, 1865, SGO, Letters Received.

50. Charles LaWall, "Report of the Pennsylvania State Pharmaceutical Association Meeting . . . Abstracts of Papers," AJP, Vol. 78 (August 1906), pp. 374-376.

51. A. K. Smith to Dunster, September 14, 1863, SGO, Letters Received. See also, "Statement of the Cost of Powders Prepared at the U.S.A. Laboratory During

the Year 1863," and "Statement of the Cost of Preparations Manufactured at the Furnace Room," in Maisch MSS.

52. Bill to Satterlee, December 31, 1864, SGO, Letters Received.

53. A. K. Smith, "Statement of cost price and market value of preparations manufactured and put up at the U.S.A. Laboratory, Philadelphia, Pa. since its commencement, March 1863, to Sept. 30, 1865," SGO, Letters Received; John M. Maisch, "Statistics of the U.S. Army Laboratory," pp. 275-278.

54. Hammond testimony, Hammond court martial trial.

55. Andrew K. Smith affidavit, June 28, 1879, Hammond ACP file.

56. *Senate Report,* No. 102, 45th Congress, 2nd Session, February 19, 1878, 14 pp.

57. MSH, Part III, Vol. I, p. 365.

58. Bill to Satterlee, December 31, 1864, SGO, Letters Received.

59. McDougall to Barnes, March 29, 1866 (fair copy), SGO, Letters Received.

60. Spencer, By Order of the Surgeon General, to Bill, December 14, 1865 (fair copy), SG Letterbooks, Military Letters.

61. Barnes to Meigs, October 15, 1863 (endorsement, fair copy), SG Letterbooks, Letters to the War Department.

62. See Chapter 2, p. 29.

63. Barnes to Stanton, September 19, 1863 (fair copy), SG Letterbooks, Letters to the Secretary of War.

64. "Prices Current," *Druggists' Circular,* Vol. 9 (June 1865), p. 110.

65. Andrew K. Smith received permission to sell on the market chemicals, such as Glauber's Salt, which were residuary products of the operations. See Spencer to Murray, March 7, 1864 (fair copy), SG Letterbooks, Military Letters; A. K. Smith to id., March 5, 1864, SGO, Letters Received.

66. Maisch pointed out that the market prices that he listed in his statistical sheets were those of "large" manufacturers who would not necessarily have furnished the medical supplies if the government had purchased them on the market; some smaller suppliers would have furnished the same items for higher cost. Maisch, "Statistics of the U.S. Army Laboratory," pp. 274-275. Andrew K. Smith also argued that the Philadelphia laboratory was saving by purchasing crude drugs in bulk; a purveyor who wished to fill a small requisition with the same drug would have paid more for it. See A. K. Smith to Dunster, September 14, 1863, SGO, Letters Received.

67. Ibid.; id. to Barnes, December 10, 1863, SGO, Letters Received. See also, Procter, "Editorial Department," AJP, Vol. 35 (July 1863), p. 375. "Morphia will also be made to an extent adequate to the wants of the whole army." This was written after Procter had visited the laboratory.

68. Barnes to Stanton, October 31, 1863 (fair copy), Surgeon General's Report Book.

69. Crane, By Order of the Surgeon General, to Murray, January 12, 1864 (fair copy), SG Letterbooks, Military Letters. Some of these supplies, however, were "very irregularly distributed."

70. Edward B. Fell, "The Pharmaceutical Department of a U.S.A. Hospital," *AJP*, Vol. 37 (March 1865), p. 112. The stockpile lasted long after the war. In 1868, the surgeon general's office declared that there was no need for it to go into the market for more drugs because it still had in storage sufficient medical supplies to last for several years. See Mears & Rockwood, Chicago, to Medical Purveyor, U.S. Army, Washington, February 3, 1868 (endorsement), SGO, Letters Received.

71. Murray to Barnes, March 5, 7, 1864, SGO, Letters Received.

72. Dunster to Murray, July 24, 1863 (fair copy), Hammond court martial trial.

73. J. R. Smith to Meylert, Medical Purveyor, Louisville, August 30, 1863 (fair copy), Hammond court martial trial.

74. Fell, "The Pharmaceutical Department of a U.S.A. Hospital," p. 110.

75. Spencer, By Order of the Surgeon General, to A. K. Smith, May 27, 1864 (fair copy), SG Letterbooks, Military Letters.

76. Id. to McDougall, February 21, March 10, 1865 (fair copies); Barnes to id., February 18, 1865 (fair copy), SG Letterbooks, Military Letters. For the large number of medical supplies carried in one of these wagons, see Appendix B.

77. Murray to Barnes, December 1, 1864, SGO, Letters Received.

78. Maisch, "Statistics of the U.S. Army Laboratory," p. 275.

79. Ellis, "The Story of a Very Old Philadelphia Drugstore," p. 67.

80. *The Rich Men of Philadelphia, Income Tax of the Residents of Philadelphia,* cited in E. Digby Baltzell, *Philadelphia Gentlemen, The Making of a National Upper Class* (Glencoe, Illinois, The Free Press, 1958), p. 108.

81. [Advertisement] "Powdering and Grinding—U.S. Steam Drug Mills," *Philadelphia North American and United States Gazette,* June 6, 1865.

82. Crane, By Order of the Surgeon General, to Murray, September 23, 1863, May 23, 1864 (fair copies); Spencer, By Order of the Surgeon General, to Satterlee (fair copies), May 24; June 23, 1864, SG Letterbooks, Military Letters.

83. *150 Years Service to American Medicine* (New York, Schieffelin and Company, 1944), pp. 41, 62.

84. [Advertisement] "Resinoids, Medical Extracts, Fluid Extracts . . . which will be carefully made with improved apparatus," *Druggists' Circular,* Vol. 9 (April 1865), p. 84.

85. For the first time, the United States Pharmacopoeia in its fifth decennial revision (1873) included glycerin as a constituent of liquid extracts. For Gordon's promotion of glycerin during the war, see Gordon, "Glycerin," *Proceedings of the American Pharmaceutical Association,* 1864, pp. 238-239; see also his article, "On Glycerin As a Substitute for Alcohol," ibid., 1865, pp. 159-160. Gordon was distributing glycerin in containers that ranged from one-pound bottles to demijohns and carboys. Tens of thousands of pounds were available at his establishment; he boasted that Cincinnati ("Porkopolis") had become the center of the American glycerin manufacturing industry. See his advertisements in *Druggists' Circular,* Vol. 7 (January 1863) p. 4, Vol. 9 (April 1, 1865), p. 84. For bromine

production by Gordon, see John Uri Lloyd, "Activities of W. J. M. Gordon," *Journal of the American Pharmaceutical Association,* Vol. 16 (June 1927), p. 549.

86. Maisch, "Report on the Drug Market," pp. 196-197; "Manufacture of Soda Ash from Cryolite in America," *Chemical News,* August 31, 1865, cited in AJP, Vol. 37 (November 1865), pp. 468-469; William Haynes, *American Chemical Industry,* Vol. 1 (New York: D. Van Nostrand, 1945-1954), pp. 285-286.

87. See Chapter 3, note 35.

88. "Report of the Committee on Membership" [Obituary Notice], *Proceedings of the American Pharmaceutical Association,* 1901, p. 47.

89. *Ninth Census,* Vol. 3, pp. 395-402.

90. Maisch to A. K. Smith, January 13, 1865, Maisch MSS.

91. Ibid.; Woodward to Maisch, November 13, 20; December 10, 1863, Maisch MSS.

92. Barnes to Stanton, March 14, 1864 (endorsement, fair copy), SG Letterbooks, Letters to the Secretary of War.

93. Crane, By Order of the Surgeon General, to Satterlee, March 25, 1864 (endorsement, fair copy), SG Letterbooks, Military Letters.

94. Maisch, "Report on the Drug Market," pp. 188-189.

95. This was particularly done with quinine, opium, and other costly drugs.

96. F. B. Nichols, "Review of the New York Markets," *Druggists' Circular,* Vol. 8 (January 1864), p. 14.

97. Ibid., Vol. 9 (January 1865), p. 19.

98. Francis B. Heitman, *Historical Register and Dictionary of the United States Army from Its Organization, September 29, to March 2, 1903,* 2 vols. (Washington, DC, Government Printing Office, 1903), Vol. 1, pp. 218, 738, 860, 894.

99. These words were spoken by Guthrie. See "Proceedings and Debates of the Fourth National Quarantine and Sanitary Convention Held in June 1860," *Druggists' Circular,* Vol. 5 (February 1861), p. 38.

100. [William Procter Jr.,] "Editorial Department," AJP, Vol. 37 (September 1865), p. 399. Procter had been far from enthusiastic when the laboratories were set up in 1863; in September 1865 he declared, "Whatever may be said about the administration of Dr. Hammond, the establishment of the Government Laboratory was certainly a move in the right direction."

101. "Correspondence: Reorganization of the Medical Staff," *The Army and Navy Journal,* Vol. 2 (August 5, 1865), p. 790.

102. [William Procter Jr.], "Editorial Department," AJP, Vol. 38 (May 1866), pp. 287-288.

103. MSH, Part III, Vol. 1, p. 965.

104. [William Procter Jr.], "Medical Purveying for the U.S. Army During the Late War," AJP, Vol. 38 (May 1866), p. 271.

Index

Hammond, William Alexander
  (continued)
  and United States Army Medical
    Department, 2
  and United States Naval
    Laboratory, success of, 24
Hartshorne, Dr., 75
Henkel, Augustus, 75
Holt, Joseph, 96
Hospital stewards, 14-16
Hyer, John Jr., 44

Ichthyocolla plaster, 80, 107-108

Jacobs, Henry H., 75
James Powder, experimentally
    produced, 63
J. H. Reed & Company, 27
John Wyeth and Brother, 22, 65-66,
    89
Johnson, Charles Beneulyn, 15

Keffer, Frederick A., 77
Kennedy, George W., 16

Larrey, Dominique-Jean, 1
Lawson, Thomas, 36
Lemberger, Joseph Lyon, 16
Letterman, Jonathan
  orders that hospital stewards be
    attached to every field
    hospital, 15
  originates supply table for the
    Army of the Potomac, 17
  and United States Army Medical
    Department, 2, 6
Lincoln, Abraham, 12
Louis XIV of France, 1
Louisville Chemical Works, 74

Maisch, John Michael
  and an American source of tartar,
    91
  career, 70-73
  as chief chemist, 33
  on chloroform manufacturing,
    105-107
  conducts tests, 65
  detects adulterations, 91-93
  on drug prices, 20
  and feasibility of manufacturing
    quinine sulfate, 97-98
  improves pharmaceutical
    processes, 78
  inventions, 88
  and medicinal spirits, 108
  Parrish, association with, 73
  and pharmaceutical botany, 89
  and the Philadelphia laboratory,
    74, 120
  and Robert Shoemaker & Co., 92
  scientific investigations, 79, 88
  Smith, Andrew K., 70
  Squibb, employed by, 41, 73
  testing crude drugs, 118
  unrecognized for his services, 119
  on whiskey and wine, 91-92
Marquand, Frank, 53
Materia Medica, on U.S. Army
    supply table, 3-4, 121-137.
    See also Drugs; Medicines
Mayer, Ferdinand F., 108-109
McCormick, Charles. *See also*
    Astoria laboratory; United
    States Army Laboratories
  and acacia, 105
  and the Astoria laboratory, 29, 43,
    44-45
  career, 40-41
McDougall, Charles
  and ether, manufacturing of, 102
  medical purveyor at Philadelphia,
    77
McKesson and Robbins, 41

Order Your Own Copy of
This Important Book for Your Personal Library!

MEDICINES FOR THE UNION ARMY
The United States Army Laboratories During the Civil War

_____ in hardbound at $69.95 (ISBN: 0-7890-0946-3)

_____ in softbound at $24.95 (ISBN: 0-7890-0947-1)

COST OF BOOKS_____

OUTSIDE USA/CANADA/
MEXICO: ADD 20%_____

POSTAGE & HANDLING_____
*(US: $4.00 for first book & $1.50
for each additional book
Outside US: $5.00 for first book
& $2.00 for each additional book)*

SUBTOTAL_____

IN CANADA: ADD 7% GST_____

STATE TAX_____
*(NY, OH & MN residents, please
add appropriate local sales tax)*

FINAL TOTAL_____
*(If paying in Canadian funds,
convert using the current
exchange rate. UNESCO
coupons welcome.)*

☐ **BILL ME LATER:** ($5 service charge will be added)
(Bill-me option is good on US/Canada/Mexico orders only;
not good to jobbers, wholesalers, or subscription agencies.)

☐ Check here if billing address is different from
shipping address and attach purchase order and
billing address information.

Signature_____

☐ **PAYMENT ENCLOSED: $**_____

☐ **PLEASE CHARGE TO MY CREDIT CARD.**

☐ Visa   ☐ MasterCard   ☐ AmEx   ☐ Discover
☐ Diner's Club   ☐ Eurocard   ☐ JCB

Account # _____

Exp. Date _____

Signature _____

Prices in US dollars and subject to change without notice.

NAME _____

INSTITUTION _____

ADDRESS _____

CITY _____

STATE/ZIP _____

COUNTRY _____ COUNTY (NY residents only) _____

TEL _____ FAX _____

E-MAIL_____

May we use your e-mail address for confirmations and other types of information? ☐ Yes   ☐ No
We appreciate receiving your e-mail address and fax number. Haworth would like to e-mail or fax special
discount offers to you, as a preferred customer. **We will never share, rent, or exchange your e-mail
address or fax number.** We regard such actions as an invasion of your privacy.

Order From Your Local Bookstore or Directly From

The Haworth Press, Inc.

10 Alice Street, Binghamton, New York 13904-1580 • USA

TELEPHONE: 1-800-HAWORTH (1-800-429-6784) / Outside US/Canada: (607) 722-5857

FAX: 1-800-895-0582 / Outside US/Canada: (607) 772-6362

E-mail: getinfo@haworthpressinc.com

PLEASE PHOTOCOPY THIS FORM FOR YOUR PERSONAL USE.

www.HaworthPress.com

BOF00